X

G E O R G

D1125481

ESCAPE FROM
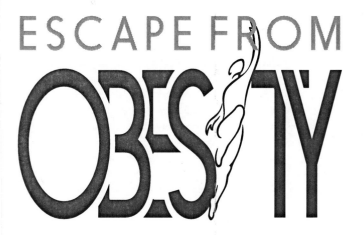
OBESITY

THE ROUTE OUT OF
THE DIET JUNGLE

**Panarc
International**

Published in Great Britain 2014 by
Panarc International Ltd.

A CIP catalogue record for this book is available
from the British Library.

Paperback ISBN 978-0-9548740-6-3

Also available as an eBook:
eBook mobi ISBN 978-0-9548740-9-4
eBook epub ISBN 978-0-9548740-7-0

Front cover image:
©istockphoto.com/londoneye

Designed at Chandler Book Design.

Printed in Great Britain by
Ingram Spark

CONTENTS

Foreword

This book is *not* another diet book. There are already hundreds of those in existence. None of them has proved very effective in preventing people from over eating, and none of them has halted the exponential rise of the obesity epidemic since the phoney war on cholesterol began in the 1950s.

All of these books have one thing in common: they all offer you one or another method of starvation. In reality nobody is prepared to spend the rest of their life starving, and these diets offer no more than a temporary diversion from the real issue. What everyone wants is very simple - to be happy with eating normal, nutritional, everyday food that gives you all the energy you need but without the extra intake that piles on the weight.

Another diet book is unnecessary. What is needed is a book about nutrition and normal human eating habits that helps overweight people to escape from obesity permanently

- a book based on pertinent facts, many of which have been long forgotten, or simply ignored, by the diet industry. Most of these facts are known but are disregarded by health professionals, health organisations and government departments. All of these facts are denied, or twisted out of existence, by the international food industry and the pharmaceutical giants worldwide.

New and dubious information has replaced many of these facts in the minds of both the population and policy makers in the Western World. The resultant obesity epidemic started about a decade or so after the Second World War ended, and now seems unstoppable, as you will see later.

However, all is not lost. Every overweight or obese person can escape this burden if they make themselves familiar with the fundamental reasons for weight gain and the measures that they can take to reverse it.

There are two features of the diet debate I would like to consider before I go into the relevant facts relating to the practical measures involved in permanent weight control.

The first is that there are many thousands of scientific papers in circulation dealing with nutrients and nutrition. The overwhelming majority of these are the results of clinical experience, painstaking research and experimentation carried out by dedicated scientists. Other published papers are based on epidemiological studies.

What is remarkable about this wealth of information is that one set of published research reports, in reputable publications, emerging from internationally recognised scientific establishments, will assert that, in nutritional terms, 'A' is, in fact, 'B'. Roughly the same number of papers will assert that 'B' is, in fact, 'A'.

Some of these assertions are supported by common sense and historical experience. Others are plainly contrived, serving group commercial interests. On a banal level they go something like this: "Wonder drug cures headaches; therefore the cause of headaches must be a lack of Wonder drug in the patient".

After reading many scientific reports, and the results of lots of epidemiological findings, I have to say I no longer find this at all amusing! The practical manifestation of all this contradictory information is familiar to everyone. We have seen in the media one day that "eggs or red wine or salt are good for you". A year or two later the same sources inform you that "you must eat no more than one egg a week, drink no more than a glass of wine a month and cut down on your salt intake". The same propaganda wave is disseminated concerning saturated animal fat, polyunsaturated fats, sugar and other carbohydrates. Not surprisingly, the population is ill informed, rudderless and confused.

Secondly, I need to say something about me. I am not a nutritionist, although I have studied the subject of nutrition and human eating habits for over 10 years. I am a writer and director of training programmes on technical developments and safety issues for the international Merchant Navy. For the past 40 years or so, I have analysed raw data, technical and scientific reports, as they related to merchant shipping, distilled them down to specific practical instructions and recommendations to educate the ever changing population of merchant seafarers globally. I have applied this analytical experience to the subject of nutrition for the last ten years.

In the course of this activity, I have co-written, directed and produced a video programme with the title: *Be Slim*

Without Dieting, which was released in 2003. My scientific advisor and co-writer was Dr. Barry Groves PhD, author of *Eat Fat, Get Thin*, *The Calorie Fallacy* and *Trick and Treat*.

Furthermore, my wife and I are blessed with a very healthy appetite. We eat well and without restriction within our means. Before 2002 that meant that my Body Mass Index was over 30; I was obese. My wife was always on a diet of some sort or another. Since 2002, when we became aware of some crucial facts about nutrition during the research period for our documentary video, we have changed our lives. We still eat what we like, but the food we now like has changed.

My wife, at 70, is now her ideal weight, while I am currently around 4-5 pounds over my optimum weight because I am a 'piggy'! But, now, I am happy with that.

Neither of us has seen a doctor for at least 20 years, except when I had to see him about an incident relating to several visits to a dentist who was obsessed with scanning my teeth on every visit. I have never been in hospital as a patient in my 76 years of eating well.

I can now give the reader an undertaking. Everything that is written in this book is in line with the current understanding of the science of nutrition and our knowledge of the requirements of the human body for natural nutrients, the nutrients that have provided the human race with a healthy diet for hundreds of thousands of years. I will present the facts in the form of an informal one-to-one discussion with you, the reader, and will present the historic/scientific background in separate sections.

The aim is to enable you to make your own choices, to decide on your own food preferences and to move away from foods that provide you with too many calories and insufficient nutrients. Without spending more money, you can choose foods that please your appetite and give you a better nutrient balance at a reduced volume of food. All this, without having to starve!

You are an individual, with your own character, likes and dislikes, strengths and weaknesses. But you have been given generalized advice by diet books, government departments and health professionals who have told you to avoid saturated fat, sugar and salt, exercise more and have a balanced diet. This so-called, 'healthy eating' advice is now, in 2014, considered by scientists, as well as many health professionals, to be the worst and most damaging health advice of the past 40 years. Why? Because it has resulted in an epidemic of heart disease, hypertension, strokes and diabetes – not to mention obesity.

Let's get back to basics. Let's establish, first of all, what is the cause of obesity. The cause of obesity is FOOD.

Now let's establish what provides the means of escape from obesity.

The means of escape from obesity is provided by FOOD.

No, it is not nonsense nor is it confusing. Read on.

Foods that cause obesity can be described as those which contain predominantly, or in some cases exclusively, energy sources over nutrients. For example, sugar in all its form, sweet fruit juices, fizzy drinks, cokes, cakes, biscuits, cereals, processed 'low fat', 'low cholesterol' and 'fat free' meals and desserts. These foods and drinks are sold to appeal to the eye and to the taste buds encouraging you to eat and drink of these much more than you actually need for your metabolic processes or to satisfy your thirst or hunger.

Foods that provide the means of escape from obesity are those which provide a much better balance between nutrients and energy and so will entirely satisfy your appetite at a significantly lower volume - for example, eggs, cheese, cream, meat, poultry, fish and wholemeal bread.

Escaping from obesity is a process by which you distinguish between foods that cause obesity and those that provide a means of escape from it. In order to distinguish between the two you need accurate information about the foods you have available to eat. That is what this book will provide.

You do not need any more advice. You need simple, honest facts about the foods you have available to eat and how they impact on your weight. You also need a proven 'roadmap' to follow, a step by step process that will suit you and that will enable you to regain your normal weight. That is also what this book will give you.

Whilst the processes of human metabolism are hugely complex and dense, the practical measures you can take in order to control your weight are surprisingly simple. But you must stop hoping for a miracle powder, pill or drink, or looking for some remedies or physical tricks that will do it for you or, unbelievably, resorting to surgical intervention. Subjecting yourself to a surgical process that gets rid of most of your stomach is wilful bodily harm, not a million miles away from curing headache with a lobotomy.

Most obese people are desperate to regain their normal weight, to escape the discomfort, the shame, the feeling of guilt and the pain. The only effective way to achieve this is for them to take control of their current eating habits.

And the only way they can do this is by becoming fully aware of the nutritional values of the foods available for them to eat and the way their bodies use these values. I know because I was one of these obese people. As you have chosen to read this book, you may also be one.

If you are overweight, if you are a parent with overweight children or, if you are an expectant mother who wishes her baby never to experience the difficulties and diseases associated with obesity, just read on.

George Bekes 2014.

1

Starting point
Reality Check 1

Here's the good news: by starting to read this book you have demonstrated your intention to escape from obesity and you are prepared to do something about it. Congratulations!

To assist you with this journey, I would like to share with you a superb tip I received years ago about the way to set out on an important task or to reach a set goal. Here it is.

Write down, yes, write down what you actually want to achieve: how much weight you want to lose to get to your normal weight and how long you would like it to take.

Bear in mind that aiming to lose more than 2-3 pounds a week is unrealistic and unhealthy and unnecessary. You are not in a race, but on a route to regain your normal weight. So, you write down your realistic goal.

Now break up the timescale you have given yourself into four periods and write down what you hope to achieve during the first period, then the second and so on.

Then, place your target plan somewhere where it is visible at all times so that you can look at it when things get a little wobbly. At times like this, and there are going to be times like this, shut your eyes and imagine that you have already achieved your desired weight loss. Imagine how you will look and feel as the new you. Imagine what you would do, what you would wear when you are your new you. Imagine how your loved ones and your friends will think about you and your achievements. Imagine the joy the health and happiness you will experience. When you open your eyes, you will say to yourself: 'Wobble, what wobble?'

I was amazed how useful this little trick turned out to be for me when trying to get something difficult and tedious done which was important to us.

Now, let's establish your starting position. This requires a few reality checks. Let's look at the reasons for the obesity epidemic that has plagued the developed world for the last half century. The official explanation is that people live a much more sedentary life than before and eat a lot of junk food.

I say, tell that to the millions of people around the globe who religiously follow the officially promoted 'healthy eating' advice and spend their spare time and cash in gyms and jogging every weekend while, much to their dismay, their weight increases. Obviously, the reasons lie elsewhere. Let's resolve this issue on the basis of 'true facts'.

There are over 100 million obese people living in developed, Western, countries and in so called emerging economies such as Brazil and China. The figure has risen continually since the late 1970s. The reason for this is beyond argument.

After the Second World War ended, world leaders as well as global health organisations started to focus on a simple question: "How can we feed the ever increasing world population in the future? How can we produce the required amount of food?" The obvious answer emerged and was rapidly accepted as official policy by the developed nations, primarily lead by the United States and Great Britain.

It went like this. There is no way that the world will be able to produce the required number of animals to provide the required amount of meat and saturated fat - the primary sources of nutrients for humanity for millions of years - to feed the world. However, with advanced agricultural methods, plenty of cereals (i.e. grains, seeds, and pulses), roots, green vegetables, berries and other types of fruit can be produced round the globe - and at a much lower cost. So, the obvious answer is, instead of feeding the animals with cereals, grass, roots and pulses, we must feed human populations directly with these food stuffs.

What politicians involved appeared to have overlooked is that the animals that have evolved to eat, and to find the required nutrients in, grass, cereals, pulses, leaves, and other foods of vegetable origin have arrived at this evolutionary stage over many hundreds of thousands of years; may be even millions of years. During this time, humans have evolved to eat primarily meat, fish and animal fat, through hunting, supplemented by wild berries, roots, nuts and fruit. The fact that we have started adding some agricultural produce to our traditional diet during the past 3000 to 5000 years is almost inconsequential because, in evolutionary terms, this is like yesterday.

The politicians failed to take into account the likelihood, if not the certainty, that a sudden change in the types of foods humans eat would have untold consequences. This is because the proposition was not to add to our traditional foods but to largely replace them with vegetable oils, starch and sugar, all of which are rather new to human metabolism.

No sooner had this idea penetrated the consciousness of policy makers worldwide, than two American doctors - John Gofman, in 1950, and later Ancel Keys, in 1953 - produced epidemiological findings that indicated that eating meat and meat products, especially saturated animal fat, was bad for our health. In particular, they associated animal fats with heart attacks due to their cholesterol content. They used different methods to come to the same proposition. Neither of those methods was ever authenticated scientifically.

This did not stop the proposition from gaining global acceptance, despite the fact that Dr. Ancel Keys himself, three years later in 1956, intimated that there was no credible evidence to show that consumed cholesterol plays a causal role in the development of heart attacks.

There is a saying that "lies will travel round the globe before truth puts its boots on". With lightning speed, the World Health Organisation, governments and health institutions embraced what is known as the Diet/Heart Hypothesis (i.e. consumed cholesterol causes heart disease) and produced, in the 1970s, the concept of "healthy eating", promoting, amongst other things, plant based oils and spreads in place of saturated animal fats. Meanwhile, the food industry started to produce 'low fat', 'fat free' and 'low cholesterol' processed foods with flavour-enhancing chemicals and elevated levels of sugar and salt.

During the next decade or two, new foods appeared on shelves, appealing to the eye and to the taste buds with little regard to the nutrients they contained. Some even contained chemical substances not considered safe for human consumption. Saturated animal fat, besides providing essential fatty acids in a healthy ratio, also gave flavour to food; these new foods had to have that flavour restored by adding salt and sugar.

All this amounted to a gigantic "laboratory" experiment where the populations in the developed world - like laboratory rats - were subjected to a vast dietary switch. Presided over by the World Health Organisation, governments and their health departments, national health services, charitable organisations, right down to your local GP, people were persuaded to replace traditional foods with new ones made up of plant based processed or refined ingredients.

Unfortunately for us laboratory rats, our weight started to increase, and the incidence of arthritis, heart disease, strokes, high blood pressure and diabetes also started to grow. These health issues were either non-existent or appeared rarely at the beginning of the 20th century but are now presenting themselves as epidemics at the beginning of the 21st century, as the population has followed the advice given to them by health professionals, by charities promoting health issues and even by government departments who are, supposedly, guardians of the nation's health.

However, the pharmaceutical industries welcomed this deterioration in the population's health and responded by producing a range of drugs designed to deal with the symptoms of these modern diseases. They developed drugs to reduce high blood pressure, reduce cholesterol, stop heartburn and deal with diabetes and arthritis, all results of eating the new foods.

But what were these new foods? They were foods

containing too much starch, sugar, trans-fats, shelf-life-increasing chemicals - and too little of the essential fatty acids, first class proteins and other nutrients required in the processes of human metabolism.

We now have a global food industry, producing trillions of dollars' worth of processed foods, providing hundreds of thousands of jobs and millions of dollars of taxes for governments. We have a global pharmaceutical industry producing trillions of dollars' worth of drugs and providing hundreds of thousands of jobs. We have health authorities and experts who have promoted the "healthy eating" doctrine for decades and we have governments that have supported it. There is no easy or immediate way back.

The good news is that *you* can escape from this entirely bizarre and tragic situation that has created many millions of overweight or obese people. It is within your power to change what made you overweight in the first place and, on the basis of real nutritional facts and a 'road map', using your own preferred foods, to regain your normal weight for ever. The facts described in this book will help you to do just that.

Always remember, since the 1950s we have been told that the foods humanity had existed on previously were bad for us. To give this some context, it is implied that mothers' milk, containing saturated animal fat, fats that your own body stores for your survival when food is in short supply, the fats that make up your own brain and fats your body cells are made of are all bad for your health. If you believe that you will believe anything!

Throughout history, there have, of course, always been fat people, just as some will be obese in the future, and there are many reasons for this, ranging from hereditary problems, or eating habits arising from psychological, emotional or health disorders. How these issues impact on your escape route from obesity will be discussed later. But for now we are concerned with the obesity problems of normal, otherwise confident, people who keep putting on weight despite the fact that they follow the prevailing 'healthy eating' advice from various, seemingly knowledgeable and certainly powerful sources.

Does this make sense to you? Billions of pounds have been spent over the last 60 years by governments, by the food and pharmaceutical industries, by charities and research organisations, on giving you advice about 'healthy eating', about the food you should eat, the food you should avoid and the best ways to control your weight. **Yet, the obesity epidemic has grown uncontrollably during the same period.**

The same 'healthy eating' advice was given to the population during the latter quarter of the 20th Century for avoiding coronary heart disease, strokes and diabetes, yet these diseases have also become increasingly prevalent, and the latest scientific thinking, supported by medical opinion, is that the 'healthy eating' advice, based on a phoney war on cholesterol, is the most serious medical error of the past 40 years.

Nevertheless, this trend is not likely to change because it is now the world wide food industry, worth many trillions of dollars, which effectively controls, one way or another, what we eat. Governments and health organisations appear to be reluctant or impotent to do anything about it.

If you want further evidence for this extraordinary state of affairs, read the New York Times report, published under the title: *The Extraordinary Science of Addictive Junk Food.*

This report is about a meeting that took place as early as the 8th April 1999 at the Minneapolis headquarters of Pillsbury where 11 company executives from Nestlé, Kraft, Nabisco, General Mills, Procter & Gamble, Coca-Cola and Mars assembled..

They discussed the obesity epidemic and how much responsibility for it rested with these giants of food manufacture. James Behnke, a chemist with a degree in food sciences and a 55-year-old executive at Pillsbury, was the host. Prior to this meeting he was engaged in conversations with food-science experts who had been painting an alarming picture about the public's ability to cope with the industry's processed foods in view of the human body's fragile controls on overeating, and in the face of some processed foods making people feel hungrier still. It was time to ask whether these companies had gone too far in creating and marketing products that posed very grave health concerns. Little or nothing has been done since 1999 to address these concerns.

Be that as it may, individuals who wish to escape from this obesity epidemic can change their own situation without hindrance. But for that to happen they need objective facts about nutrition and the food that is available for consumption today.

This book provides these facts for you. Everything you read here has been distilled from scientific knowledge that was disseminated in respected and generally peer-reviewed scientific literature.

I do not add anything to it. I do not give advice here of any sort. No medical advice, no nutritional advice. For medical advice you need to consult your own doctor. I simply present you with reliable, factual information about nutrition and a route map to help you along the way to achieve your normal weight.

I will, however, share with you some of my own relevant personal experiences which, I hope, will enable you avoid some of the mistakes I made along the same escape route. When I offer these personal observations, please take them as merely my comments on the issues to which they relate.

I repeat, it is not advice you need but nutritional knowledge in order to create your own preferred eating habits that will help you escape from your own pains and suffering resulting from being overweight. It is for you to decide how you are going to benefit from the facts I include in the book. This is a joint project. I will do my part.

If you are interested in the scientific/historic background to the above developments, here it is:

At the beginning of the 20th Century, a Russian physiologist, Anitschkov, first voiced a view that cholesterol in the blood is the cause of atherosclerosis. He came to this conclusion after feeding rabbits with very high doses of cholesterol after which he detected blocked arteries in those rabbits.

Dr. John Gofman, an American doctor, came up with the same hypothesis, in 1950, namely, that the presence of cholesterol in the blood may be responsible for the development of atherosclerosis, leading to heart attack. He came to this conclusion after more or less repeating the experiments of Dr. Anitschkov.

These two good men completely ignored the fact that rabbits never eat animal fat high in cholesterol. This substance is completely alien to their metabolism.

(Similar mistaken approaches are evident in science all the time!)

Following this episode, another American doctor, the aforementioned Ancel Keys came to a similar conclusion, in 1953, after conducting an epidemiological study, relating the rate of mortality from Coronary Heart Disease to the level of consumption of saturated animal fats in certain countries. Six countries to be precise. (In some circles this is called the "seven country" study which was, in fact, a follow up study).

Two things need to be emphasised about Dr. Ancel Keys' findings. He studied the data available in 22 countries, but chose only six of them which could be linked together with a more or less "straight line" on a graph, indicating a correlation between death from CHD and the consumption rate of saturated animal fat. The other important factor about Dr. Ancel Key's work is that he did not use the level of consumption of saturated animal fats at all in those six countries but the amount of fat AVAILABLE for consumption. The Diet/Heart Hypothesis was born based on this dubious and vacuous evidence.

An even more telling event emerged regarding Dr Ancel Keys' activities when, in 1954, the recently formed World Health Organisation created its first Expert Committee on the Pathogenesis of Atherosclerosis to discuss the growing epidemic of coronary heart disease and heart attacks. The seminar was held in Geneva. Among world luminaries of medical science was Ancel Keys who spoke about his diet-heart–cholesterol hypothesis. In mid-flight he was interrupted by a George Pickering, a Knight of the Realm, who asked Dr Keys to produce a single piece of evidence which supported his hypothesis. Dr Keys, as the story goes, plucked one out of thin air which was immediately demolished by the distinguished listeners.

Having left Geneva, Dr. Keys set about organising a study to provide evidence for his hypothesis. That is how he contrived what is now referred to as the Seven Countries Study. It was immediately evident that the seven countries were very carefully selected to provide the evidence he sought.

It has to be said that for the following two decades numerous studies were carried out and promoted by various US government departments and organisations, such as the American Heart Association, their British counterpart, and the Framingham Study that started in 1948 - to name a few. All produced reports that seemed initially to support Dr. Keys' hypothesis about the connection between blood cholesterol and CHD. But that support began to diminish as time went by.

Be that as it may, the so called "diet/heart hypothesis" became well established without the benefit of concrete evidence, despite strenuous efforts to find such evidence in order to silence the doubting scientists.

For example, in 1988, the Surgeon General's office in the USA decided to gather together all the evidence and produce a report to support the diet/heart hypothesis with concrete scientific evidence. Eleven years later, they abandoned their search and any plan to publish a report.

It must be noted also that one of the world's largest studies, the Framingham Heart Study, could NOT confirm the causal link between elevated serum cholesterol and Coronary Heart Disease. In a report, published 30 years after the study commenced, they concluded that only an elevated level of serum cholesterol could be considered a risk factor of CHD; one amongst many others, such as, smoking, obesity, high blood pressure and psychological stress.

Despite all this, the "healthy eating" advice, based on the diet/heart hypothesis, has formed the basis of the official "wilful bodily harm" that governments and health organisations, aided and abetted by the food industry, have meted out to millions of obese people the world over. This is in the face of statements made by Dr. Ancel Keys himself, in 1956, and as late as 1997, that there is no connection between cholesterol in food and the level of serum cholesterol. By implication, dietary cholesterol in the blood should not, as such, be considered as a possible cause of CHD.

Today, we still have the official "Healthy Eating" advice, wholly based on an unproven and confusing epidemiological study conducted in the middle of the last Century.

Among many scientists and doctors who have lifted the lid off the 'healthy eating" advice, based on the Diet/Heart Hypothesis, is Dr. Sylvan Lee Weinberg, former President of the American College of Cardiology, former President of the American College of Chest Physicians and editor of the American Heart Hospital Journal, who in 2004, issued a critique in a paper:

"The low-fat, Diet/Heart hypothesis – has been controversial for nearly 100 years. The low fat, high-carbohydrate diet, promulgated vigorously... may well have played an unintended role in the current epidemics of obesity, lipid abnormalities,

type II diabetes and metabolic syndromes. This diet can no longer be defended by appeal to the authority of prestigious medical organisations or by rejecting clinical experience and a growing medical literature suggesting that the much maligned low-carbohydrate, high-protein diet may have a salutary effect on the epidemics in question".

Later publications of research results and clinical experience also support the view that the prevailing "healthy eating" advice causes untold harm within the population.

Much more information is available on:

www.pubmed.org
www.thincs.org
www.second-opinions.co.uk
www.drpeeke.com

2

About The Healthy Eating Advice

Reality Check 2

The next step in preparation for the journey is to understand how we have developed our eating habits under the rules of the spurious "healthy eating" advice, promoted officially during the past forty or so years. What did they tell us, in the context of weight control?

* avoid saturated animal fat, sugar and salt
* use complex carbohydrates for your energy sours
* consume polyunsaturated fat instead of butter
* exercise more
* have a balanced diet

This was clear advice from government, the National Health Service, health professionals, your own GP and scientific establishments. There was no reason to question the validity and authenticity of such clear advice. Now, however, in the light of new research and clinical evidence, there are plenty of reasons to question this vacuous advice. It is very important to understand why this advice is *wrong*, leaving to one side for now the empirical evidence that it has proved to be entirely counterproductive.

The advice to avoid saturated animal fat arises from the mistaken belief held in the middle of the 20th Century that the cholesterol contained in animal fat, if consumed, could lead to heart disease. We have already dealt with this phoney war on cholesterol that ended up depriving populations of one of the most valuable, traditional, foods for human consumption. We will deal with this most important issue in greater detail later.

The advice to avoid sugar and salt turns out to be the most ironic because the flavour of modern processed, manufactured foods that contain little or no saturated fat would not appeal to the consumers' taste buds without the addition of large amounts of sugar and salt. The case for avoiding sugar would have been helpful but for its elevated use in processed packaged foods and soft drinks. Sugar provides 'empty calories: i.e. energy without any nutrients. To add insult to injury, high fructose corn syrup (HFCS) was added to virtually all processed foods and drinks. The syrup is not only much sweeter than sugar, but is also an industrial product that poisons the liver causing the entire range of diseases listed under the group name Metabolic Syndrome. More will be said about HFCS later.

The advice to avoid salt is based on the belief that over consumption of salt can lead to hardening of the arteries and elevated blood pressure, working on the basis that the body's water and salt equilibrium is very accurately controlled. In reality, high consumption of salt simply results in the excess salt being excreted. Low consumption of salt, lower than the body requires, results in muscle cramp among other electrolyte complications and, eventually, death.

Advising the consumption of complex carbohydrates instead of saturated fat as the recommended source of energy is curious in the face of advice to consume less sugar which is itself a simple carbohydrate. All carbohydrates or starches, such as cereals, seeds, roots, green vegetables and fruits and all foods made from them, when metabolised, end up as glucose in the blood, just as sugar does, except in twice the volume that sugar produces. Sugar produces one part glucose and one part water. Complex carbohydrates produce two parts of glucose. Although they contain some protein, vitamins and fibre (often termed roughage), they are mostly empty calories. Any excess consumption of energy from these starches, if not used promptly by the metabolic processes, is stored as fat in the body. This does not happen when saturated fat is consumed for energy.

The advice of using polyunsaturated, plant based, fat in place of saturated animal fat is even more inexplicable in the eyes of scientists today. There are two reasons why. One, they can only be safely used when cold. Once heated, they break down into their components, including trans-fats, a well-known precursor of cancer. Two, spreadable, hydrogenated versions such as margarines are full of chemical residues from the manufacturing processes and are highly detrimental to health. Continual irritation causes inflammation of the artery walls leading to cholesterol build up to protect the tissues. This is now recognised as the most relevant risk factor regarding the development of CHD. And this, of course, is the very development which the promoters of the 'healthy eating' advice set out to avoid. (See fuller explanation of this very important process later when I give the historic/scientific background.)

The advice to exercise more is beneficial for two reasons. First, exercise speeds up metabolic processes. Secondly, exercise reduces tensions and triggers extra beneficial hormone activity. However, as a method of weight control it is of limited value.

Now we come to the most banal part of the advice: 'have a balanced diet'. If a person follows exactly the 'healthy eating' advice and has a breakfast of cereals with skimmed milk and sugar, followed by a piece of toast with jam, then has a cup of coffee with biscuits mid-morning, followed by a lunch consisting of a sandwich and another at tea time followed by a dinner of potatoes, pasta or rice, vegetables, and a piece of lean meat or fish, how on Earth will that person be able to balance the intake of all that starchy food?

So much more could be said about the official 'healthy eating' advice given to the population for the past half century. Even more disturbing is the fact that in October 2013 the prominent food manufacturers agreed with the British government to cut down on the saturated fat content of their products. What a complete nutritional farce that is, in the light of modern science!

If you are interested in the scientific/historic background to the above developments, here it is:

_____

"For a modern disease to be related to an old-fashioned food is one of the most ludicrous things I have ever heard" Dr. T. L. Cleave

"There are three ways in which a substance can increase the risk of cancer: it can cause body cells to

become cancerous; it can promote a cancer's growth; it can suppress the immune system. Polyunsaturated vegetable oils have been shown to do all three."
Dr. Barry Groves

Polyunsaturated vegetable oils contain large levels of linoleic acid which was used in the early days of spare part surgery to suppress the immune system to prevent rejection. Its use was abandoned when it was suspected of causing cancer. In contrast, scientists at the Department of Surgical Oncology, Roswell Park Cancer Institute as well as the Department of Biochemistry and Molecular Biology, New Jersey Medical School, found that Conjugated Linoleic Acid in the diet protects against several cancers. The best sources of Conjugated Linoleic Acid are kangaroo fat, dairy products or the fat on red meat, particularly beef.

Of all the factors in our modern world that are working against our immune defences, our diet is the worst, for this is exactly what happens if we eat too much carbohydrate, in particular, too much sugar.

Example:

- *Caramel Frappuccino with whipped cream 270cal, 11 tsp of sugar,*

- *Original coca cola (330ml) 139cal, 9 tsp of sugar,*

- *Regular Pepsi cola (330ml) 142cal, 9tsp of sugar,*

- *Mars Bar (51gr) 230cal. 8tsp of sugar,*

Right back in the period between the 1950s to the 1970s Professor John Yudkin, former Professor of Physiology at Queen Elisabeth College, University of London, former Professor of Nutrition and Diet, had warned against the detrimental effects of consuming sugar. He was in direct opposition to the Diet/Heart hypothesis which started the 'phoney war' on dietary cholesterol. He published a book "PURE, WHITE AND DEADLY" in which he described exactly the harm sugar represents to human health. Now, in the first decade of the 21st Century, several doctors, scientists and politicians pretend that they have suddenly discovered the harmful nature of sugar and compared it to that of tobacco.

Professor Yudkin referred to honey, too. Honey metabolizes exactly as sugar does. Yet there is a considerable difference between eating sugar and honey. There are two reasons for this. One, humanity consumed honey for at least 8000-10,000 years according to the evidence, and probably in fact a lot longer. Consequently, human metabolism has evolved to utilize honey. Secondly, raw honey contains complex array of compounds, such as macronutrients and micronutrients, enzymes, probiotics and prebiotics. Sugar (sucrose) was introduced to the human diet only in the 1800s and contains no nutrients.

A research team writing in the Journal of the American Medical Association says: "It may be stated categorically, that the storage of fat, and therefore the production and maintenance of obesity, cannot take place unless glucose is being metabolised. Since glucose cannot be used by most tissues without the presence of insulin, it also may be stated categorically that obesity is impossible in the absence of adequate tissue concentration of insulin...."

Thus, an abundant supply of carbohydrate food exerts a powerful influence in directing the stream of glucose metabolism into lipogenesis, whereas a relatively low carbohydrate intake tends to minimize the storage of fat"

America's leading cardiovascular research scientist Dr James DiNicolantonio argues that guidance for the past 60 years has been "deeply flawed" and that diets low in saturated fat do not prevent heart disease or improve health.

He wants health warnings to be issued over sugar, which is now included in everyday foods, meaning people are now unwittingly consuming record amounts. "A change in these recommendations is drastically needed as public health could be at risk," he said.

British cardiologist Dr Aseem Malhotra says the public could just as effectively protect themselves from heart disease by eating butter, milk and cheese in moderation and adopting the Mediterranean diet. Dr DiNicolantonio said the rise in diabetes and obesity correlated with the increase in carbohydrate consumption.

He added: "There is no conclusive proof that a low-fat diet has any positive effects. The literature indicates a general lack of any effect (good or bad) from a reduction in fat intake.

"The public fear that saturated fat raises cholesterol is completely unfounded; [it] is worsened when fat is replaced with carbohydrate."

The best way to avoid heart problems was a diet low in refined carbohydrates, sugars and processed foods.

The greatest danger to human health is represented by the addition – since the early 1980s - of high fructose corn syrup to virtually all manufactured food products, fruit juices and other soft drinks. Since the early 2000s many scientists and doctors focused on the detrimental effects of consuming high fructose corn syrup. Among them Robert H. Lustig, an American paediatric endocrinologist at the University of California, San Francisco (UCSF) where he is a Professor of Clinical Paediatrics. He was among the people who publicised the fact – as every biochemist knows - that high fructose corn syrup can only be metabolised in the liver, unlike sucrose or glucose, which means that the brain is not receiving any signal that energy was consumed, or that what was consumed was sufficient for the body's need for energy. Also, the impact on the health of the liver of high fructose corn syrup is almost identical to that of Ethanol. In fact, high fructose corn syrup acts as poison in the body. It is the main cause of metabolic syndrome, that is, a disorder of energy utilization and storage, diagnosed by a co-occurrence of the following medical conditions: obesity, elevated blood pressure, elevated fasting plasma glucose, high serum triglycerides, type 2 diabetes and low high-density cholesterol (HDL) levels.

Much more information is available on:
www.pubmed.org
www.thincs.org
www.second-opinions.co.uk
www.drpeeke.com

3

Your Current Eating Habits
Reality Check 3

When is a person overweight or obese? This is a question that scientists and health professionals have been arguing for a long time. And there are many different answers, some based on science, some based on 'ideal' considerations.

Most are expressed in a number of published tables, for example, the Body Mass Index which compares height with weight, the stipulated correct waist measurements for men and women, or measuring the thickness of fat under the skin. These methods are familiar to all of us. But, as we are all different from one another, isn't it a waste of time trying to decide which 'ideal' applies to any one individual?

I believe that your personal ideal weight is what you want it to be. In this context, are you overweight or obese? If yes, read on. You need to know what you are doing that makes you fat before you can create your own plan for reducing your weight.

And then you must decide that you definitely want to escape *permanently* from being overweight or obese.

This is an entirely different process from dieting to lose a few pounds before a wedding or a holiday. What should help you in taking this decision is the knowledge that you may also escape from some weight-related health issues, such as, arthritis, heart disease, diabetes, high blood pressure, joint pains and so on, or prevent them from becoming a problem for you. In other words, what you will be doing is taking a life changing decision.

Making this decision is an emotional as well as an intellectual process, depending on your personal motivations and the circumstances that led you to become overweight. Following up on such a decision is not always going to be easy and will require a degree of determination.

The difficulty may arise from the fact that you may or may not be aware of all the implications involved. You might believe that you simply like to eat. You might believe that you like certain foods and that eating them gives you pleasure and comfort and you tend to lose control over them. You may even believe that you are heavy boned or your metabolism is different from others.

Besides, you hate feeling hungry. You are not alone. Right from birth, we all learn very quickly that food gives us a sense of pleasure, comfort, safety and satisfaction and the lack of food engenders in us the feeling of discomfort, hunger, fear and pain. Of course, all of the above may play a part in making your decision to address your weight issue.

You must do your own heart searching about this, as your very first vital step, if you wish to escape from being overweight. When you have a full awareness of the reasons for consuming the kind and quantity of food that have caused your obesity, you will be able to make the changes that will enable you, along the way, to regain your target weight.

Take your time. It is more important for you to understand the way to proceed to permanent weight loss rather than to achieve an immediate but temporary weight loss. Unfortunately, there is a popular conception, created by the many hundreds of dieting books, that, if you just follow their various recommendations you will lose weight for ever. This is unfortunate for two main reasons.

First, following the recommendations in dieting books leads to starvation and, when you stop starving and return to your usual diet, you will put the pounds back and more. The second reason is that the dieter stays uninformed about the reasons for being obese; that is, what it is in their normal eating habits that makes them fat.

Taking control of your eating habits, based on nutritional information, is a completely different process. You know what to do, and why, in order to escape from obesity permanently. Once you have started the process the kilos will drop off soon enough. You are also likely to continue with the process because you will do it without experiencing hunger and you will discover new flavours and develop the taste for a greater variety of food along the way. You will delight in eating food without feeling guilty and begin to enjoy life again.

Now, you need to look first at your relationship with food in general and at the eating pattern you follow daily.

Most of us become emotionally involved with food right from birth. As adults, we no longer just feed ourselves to provide the nutrients and the energy we need for our metabolic functions. Rather, we enjoy the pleasure of eating our favourite dishes, of having breakfast, lunch and dinner and other things besides, regardless of our actual requirement for energy and nutrients. We have developed a liking for certain foods because of their appeal to our taste buds and our eyes. We pay little attention to their energy content or nutritional value. We simply enjoy eating them. This applies equally to what we drink too. All of us are like that.

Food manufacturers know this. They use this human propensity in order to sell us many things that look good, taste great and are, therefore, 'moreish'! This has everything to do with providing you with the pleasure of eating. They produce processed foods to satisfy and appeal to the widest consumer tastes.

As such, most of the things that food manufacturers now create for us to eat and drink today did not exist 70-80 years ago, certainly not in the form in which they are now advertised and sold to us. These artificial meals and products are created continually after many blind tasting trials and exercises. Only the meals that pass with flying colours will be found on supermarket shelves. Critically, these foods are tested on the basis of their taste and visual appeal and seldom on their nutritional value. And, as they are labelled 'low fat', 'fat free' or 'low cholesterol' we buy them as we continue to be told that these are the foods that are good for our health.

Latest research refers to a new understanding of food addiction related to the appearance of hyper palatable manufactured foods. These foods contain a *specific* combination of plant based fats, salt and sugar that impact on the reward centre in the frontal lobe of our brains – the Bliss Point - as they like to call it in America. Laboratory experiments show that the consumption of refined sugar has a pleasure sensor reaction similar to that of cocaine and morphine. The brain eventually reacts to these stimuli by diminishing the sensitivity to sugar. As a result, we have to consume more and more sugar to achieve the same pleasure sensation level. That is a major factor in weight gain if you have developed a sweet craving.

The next reality check you need to make before starting on your journey is to consider your own pattern of eating. This is very important because of its impact on your digestive processes and the efficiency of nutrient absorption in your body. You need consciously to observe and realise the following important behaviour issues.

Do you take breakfast? If you do, is it a quick bowl of sweetened cereal, topped with skimmed milk and rushed down as you head for the front door? Or, is it a more substantial, nutrient rich, morning meal?

- Do you have "elevenses"?
- Do you have a midday meal?
- Do you have snacks?
- Do you have an evening meal?
- Do you have a late night snack?
- What are your regular or favourite snacks and drinks?
- How quickly do you eat?

When you take food, do you concentrate on eating or get preoccupied with other things, such as watching television, working at your computer or reading a book or paper?

All of these questions relate to familiar habits that we have developed over time and the answers can have decisive effects on how well you will do on the way to regaining your normal weight. I will explain how these habits influence your progress. At the end of this chapter you can read some of the scientific evidence, if you are interested.

Let's start with breakfast

The story is familiar. Most of us like to stay in bed as long as possible in the morning, not wanting to face the day. One wit coined the phrase: "Good Morning…let the stress begin!"

That means, inevitably, rushing to get ready to go out. It also means that there is no time for breakfast or just about enough time for pouring some cereal into a bowl with a drop of milk and a sprinkling of sugar and throwing this down as quickly as possible. Some of us even develop the very bad habit of skipping breakfast altogether. One often hears it said: "I cannot stand the thought of food early in the morning".

The result is that normal metabolic functions are upset because some of the digestive juices, thickened during the night, are unused. Moreover, by just having a quick bowl of cereal or not having anything at all for breakfast, you also upset the energy provision for the body – right at the start of the day - in one of two ways.

In the case of the bowl of cereal, or any other sugary or starchy food (including muesli, thought to be a healthy version because of the dried fruit and nuts it contains), a sudden spike of glucose is created in the blood stream, followed by a rush of insulin to clear it all out and turn the glucose into body fat. [*Only a very small amount of glucose is tolerated in the bloodstream at any given time.*] Once that happens, there remains no source of energy in the bloodstream and hunger sets in.

In the case of having no breakfast at all the body is not provided with any energy or nutrients at all at the time when they are most needed, at the outset of the day.

Most dieticians will tell you that breakfast is the most important meal of the day. It must do two things. It must suit the functioning of your digestive system by providing the required nutrients to assist the many hormones involved in doing their jobs properly; secondly, it must provide you with an efficient source of energy to fuel your metabolic processes and keep you free of hunger until your next meal at lunch time.

For example, if you have a two-egg omelette, cooked in butter, with one piece of wholemeal buttered toast and a cup of tea, without sugar, you will avoid all the problems listed above and, at the same time, you will have sufficient energy until lunch time. You have also provided your body with a greater range of nutrients than if you had simply eaten some cereal and skimmed milk or a piece of fruit.

You can have all these required benefits for little extra cost and preparing such a breakfast will take only a few minutes more of your time. That will be recompensed by actually enjoying the meal and leaving home with a sense of satisfaction.

A special mention of the traditional cooked English breakfast should be made here. This meal provides more than enough nutrients and energy sources for one meal. If you like this breakfast, as I do, there are a large amount of empty calories that can be discarded from it without impairing the enjoyment of this world famous breakfast.

For example, if you omit the baked beans and the fried bread but have the bacon, the eggs, the sausage and the black pudding, with tomatoes and mushrooms, you will have the fat, protein and carbohydrate in the right proportions because the sausage and the black pudding will contain enough cereal to accompany the protein and the fat components. You will also have consumed some vitamins, minerals and trace elements that your body requires. At the same time, you will have prevented yourself from consuming about a third of the unnecessary calories in the meal, especially if you skip the toast.

Do you have "elevenses"?

A cup of coffee or tea mid-morning is usually very welcome especially if no breakfast has been taken. Do you take sugar in your drink? A biscuit or two, or nine, often accompanies the beverage. If you do this regularly you are effectively filling your digestive system with sugar and starch. Another glucose spike and insulin rush is on its way. Every time this happens, you run the risk of putting weight on, as the insulin deals with the excess glucose in your blood by storing it as fat in what is called adipose tissue, thus continuing a daily process that will increase your weight.

If you understand the process and keep it in mind, this is a clear point at which you can start taking control. I will say more about that later.

Do you have a midday meal?

Whether or not you have had breakfast, a midday meal is another important source of energy and nutrients. How much and in what proportions depends on what you choose to have for lunch. Again, you can choose to have a meal rich in starches and sugar, involving sandwiches, cakes, biscuits, crisps, fruit and soft drinks, creating another glucose spike. Or you can choose to have a ham or cheese salad or hardboiled eggs followed by a cup of tea or coffee. In later chapters I give specific information to help you choose meals that you will enjoy while avoiding the series of glucose spikes that propels the process of weight gain.

It is interesting to note that there are diverse views and habits existing in various parts of the world about the midday meal. For example, in the UK, most people who are at work regularly take a light meal, during half of the lunch hour. In France and in other Mediterranean countries, lunch is considered to be the main meal of the day and usually involve 2-3 courses of food. There are a number of reasons for this, mainly arising from their geographical situation and the prevailing weather patterns which created the culture of 2-hour lunches. It is a great excuse to keep out of the midday sun!

Do you have afternoon snacks?

What, if anything, do you take with your afternoon cup of tea? Taking the tea or coffee mid-afternoon is helpful if for no other reason than to maintain your fluid intake, despite the fact that these beverages are diuretic. If you have had an adequate midday meal you should not feel the need to eat anything at this point. If you do, an increase in the midday meal components may avoid your desire to have another biscuit, or nine, at this point. Reaching for a coke or other fizzy drinks at this stage means consuming several spoonsful of sugar or high fructose corn syrup with the water they contain. Sugar is without any nutrients; calories are all it contains.

Do you have an evening meal?

As far as weight control is concerned, it is the evening when you begin to wind down and your requirement for energy is gradually subsiding. Despite that, most of us have developed a social and personal habit of having the largest meal of the day at dinner. Whether or not you have a glass of your chosen alcohol with this meal, if dinner is your main meal of the day, you are more or less guaranteed to put weight on during the next 10 hours of rest.

This is the time to ensure, if you want to take control of your weight, that whatever you eat or drink in the evening will have maximum nutritional value with minimal energy component. You will see later how this can be accomplished. *[I will provide some appetising menus at the end of the book to give you this kind of dinner.]*

This applies equally to late night snacks. Do you raid the fridge and grab a piece of cheese or do you grab the biscuit tin and demolish its content while you are watching television? Do you follow that by 'inadvertently' chewing on a bar of chocolate, helping it down with a bottle of fizzy drinks? If you do any of these things you are attacking your body with the biggest glucose spike of the day, followed by the biggest insulin dump in your bloodstream. In one sitting, you may have consumed between 10 and 30 spoonsful of sugar. This is probably the most dangerous moment for your weight control. Ideally, late night snacks should be done away with. Certainly, I would pay the most close and immediate attention to this, right from the start. If you can do that, you will help your digestive system and your metabolic processes at the same time.

Now that we have briefly touched upon what you consume during the course of a day, the next thing to check is how you have your meals. What habits have you developed which may contribute to the malnutrition that you need to tackle?

We have developed a very bad habit of eating on the move or inattentively. This usually means eating quickly while our minds are on other things such as watching our favourite television drama or reality programmes. This habit impacts very badly on the efficiency of food absorption into the bloodstream.

Even more important, eating quickly and not paying attention to the food tends to interfere with a natural control mechanism we all have that controls our appetite, in particular, the signal that it sends when we have had sufficient nourishment. This control mechanism is in our brain and is referred to as the appetite centre or, as some American scientists call it, the "appestat". This appestat is intended to control accurately the intake of energy in relation to the body's energy requirements at any given time. Put in another way, the appestat attempts to balance the energy intake in food with the energy that the body actually needs at the time.

It sends a signal which means that you have had sufficient food intake for your needs, meaning that you can now stop eating. If you used up more energy one day, for example, cutting up fire wood in the garden or running a marathon, the appestat would allow you to take in more energy to compensate for such activity before it signals that you have had enough to eat. Of course, the converse is also true. During a sedentary day the appestat signals earlier that you have had sufficient food for your needs.

Unfortunately, since we have introduced a whole range of foods relatively new to our digestive processes, mainly sugar and starch, the appestat has not been able to perform accurately because it did not recognise the energy level provided by some of these foods. Some food additives, such as high fructose corn syrup, metabolise in the liver alone and send no signal at all to the brain of any kind.

Also, the digestion process of starches starts in the mouth when saliva is mixed with the food whilst chewing it. If not enough time is allowed for this to take place, the digestive process is going to be inadequate, misleading the appestat yet again.

The problem is made worse for us by eating too quickly for the appestat to react in time. Aggravated further by not paying attention, through habit, to any signal the appestat eventually manages to send.

It is, therefore, very important to give enough time for each meal to be consumed slowly while allowing our senses to be fully engaged with the sight, smell and flavour of the food.

All that I have just said about the functioning of the appestat applies to people who are on, or near their normal weight. In the case of those who are overweight or obese the functioning of the appetite centre in the brain is far less effective. The reason for this is the diminished effect of the hormones called Leptins. These hormones are produced by the fat cells in the body and their normal function is to send the message to the brain that the body is sated – no more food should be consumed. In the body of obese people unfortunately this signal gets blocked. The state of obesity is considered medically to be a chronic state of inflammation. In this state, the message created by Leptins is severely weakened if not blocked altogether. (*The scientific description of the function of Leptins is given later.*)

We now come to the most critical assessment you will need to make at the outset of your journey. If you get this right, your efforts will be well rewarded and soon. This assessment is the answer to the question: How much food and drink do you actually consume in a day? And by 'how much?', I mean all of it!

Several dieticians maintain that most people underestimate the amount of food they consume, primarily because they do not remember all the things they actually put in their mouths.

This is a problem. It really is necessary for you to absorb all the knowledge of all the components of the weight issue, if you are to arrive at the right solutions for success. Dieticians and research workers who were involved in experiments about this question all observed that the people who were least successful about listing the food they consumed in a day were people who were overweight or obese. If you want to succeed in taking control of your weight and escape from obesity, you need to know (to be accurate and honest about) your food consumption right at the outset.

To say that people who are obese simply eat too much is only partially true. In the sense that they consume more energy than they need, the commonly held view is beyond dispute. But they may not eat too much in the sense of volume of food. Obesity can be caused by eating food that is predominantly made up of starch, sugar, salt and hydrogenated, plant based and polyunsaturated fat. Look around in any supermarket today and the shelves are packed with these foods. Most breakfast cereals, pizzas, cakes, biscuits, 'low fat', 'fat free' or 'low cholesterol' processed, and packaged meals fall into this category.

You do not need to eat too much of these foods to be obese. If your food intake is made up mainly of these manufactured products, you are likely to create a constant cycle of glucose spikes and insulin dumps resulting in the energy content of the food being stored in your body as fat, while, at the same time, you will feel hungry soon after eating. This will encourage you to eat more, probably of the same things.

This leads neatly to the next question: Do you leave what you consume by way of nutrients in the hands of food manufacturers or would you rather take control of what you put into your mouth and create your own meals?

Before you take the view that you do not have time to cook for yourself because you have a lifestyle which leaves you little time for shopping or cooking, consider this: time keeps coming and it is up to you what you do with it. What is more important for you? Is what you are doing now more important than your health and weight? Would you consider changing your normal time schedule so that you have time to choose what you buy in the way of food? Would you rather create your own meals from your own chosen ingredients? The answers to these questions may have a huge impact on the success or failure of your efforts to control your weight and in your chances of escaping from obesity. Time, or its management, surely, cannot be a deciding factor when it comes to your health and well-being.

If you are interested in the scientific/historic background to the above issues, here it is:

Many scientific papers have been published containing the known reasons for people overeating and becoming obese besides the usual "sedentary life style" argument. Experiments were wide ranging, covering the physical, psychological and emotional aspects of seeking "comfort" in food.

Typical findings included a woman in her late 30s, weighing 12 stone, who suffered the loss of her young daughter. Within a very short space of time her weight went up to 19 stone, an increase of more than 100 pounds. Several studies pointed to cases of people who suffered the consequences of a divorce, loss of job, fear of financial ruin and a serious medical diagnosis. Fear and a sense of insecurity lies behind a considerable number of cases of obesity.

In one experiment doctors interviewed over 1000 obese patients at a slimming clinic to find out what sort of food they missed most during their attempt to lose weight? They have found that the overwhelming majority confessed to missing: chocolate, cakes, biscuits, ice-cream, pasta and pizza. That is to say, foods that are predominantly made up of starch and sugar prepared with plant based polyunsaturated fats. Clearly, these are the foods that had made these people obese.

A scientific experiment was carried out to check the persistence of addiction to sugar and sweetness.

If the adrenal glands are removed from rats, they drink salty water rather than pure or sweetened water due to the fact that salty water relieves the effect of the lack of adrenaline hormones. But if, before the operation, the rats are given sweetened water to drink, then, after the operation, they will choose to drink the sweetened water despite the fact that this is hugely detrimental to their health.

In one experiment several overweight women were asked to list all the food they had consumed in a week. Once that was done, the women were taken to hospital and, under controlled conditions, were given exactly the same food that they had included in the list. They all lost on average half a pound of weight per day!

Leptin is an example of a 16 Kda protein hormone that is produced in the fat cells of the body. Leptin plays a part in the regulation of body weight by interaction with the hypothalamus.

First discovered during the latter part of the 20th century, Leptin uses the bloodstream to travel into the brain. From there, Leptin is able to work on specific neurons within the hypothalamus to aid in appetite regulation. The stimulation of the hypothalamus by the Leptin usually results in sending out signals that let the body know there is currently no hunger, and it is time to refrain from the consumption of food. Because the hormone acts to control the rate and degree of hunger that the body experiences, it plays a valuable role in helping to minimize the physical desire for food, although Leptin has no impact on the emotional craving for sweets and other forms of food.

In overweight people, the Leptin produced by the body does not work properly, making the processes of weight loss and weight maintenance much more difficult. This is because of the state of chronic inflammation. Increased consumption of phytonutrients does help to fight the inflammation that causes Leptin resistance. Two types of phytonutrients commonly found in fruits and vegetables are carotenoids and flavonoids. These fat-soluble compounds work to reduce the inflammation that blocks Leptin.

Some foods, such as cherries, pomegranate, blueberries, citrus fruits and purple grapes contain the most flavonoids, but they can also be found in dark chocolate, onions and green tea. Foods such as tomatoes, broccoli, carrots, and papaya are rich in carotenoids.

A leading campaigner in the USA, Dr Pamela Peeke, MD. MPH. FACP., has been researching the impact of refined sugar on the brain and how food addiction develops. She and other scientists have realised that the consumption of sugar creates the same impact on the brain as cocaine and heroin. Dr. Peeke is also a leading figure promoting the science of Epigenetics where the impact of food intake is studied as it modifies the functioning of DNA.

Much more information is available on:
www.drpeeke.com
www.pubmed.org
www.thincs.org
www.second-opinions.co.uk

4

Creating a road map

I hope by now you have completed your truly honest food diary and the examination of your own eating habits. *[If you have children with a weight problem, the same examination should be carried out with them.]*

Now you can begin to create your own ways to reduce or eliminate, one by one, the elements that are most detrimental to your weight control. But if you are not entirely honest with your examination of your eating habits, your efforts to escape from obesity are not likely to succeed or, if they do succeed, success will come only with greater effort and may take a lot longer than necessary.

As soon as you have completed your reality checks, you are ready to get going with your escape from obesity. Rather than giving you general advice about procedure, it may be more helpful to you to have a look at how my wife and I have gone through the same process and what solutions we have chosen to escape from obesity or, in our case, regain our target weight.

This does not mean that you have to follow our example. You are a different person from us, with different habits, different preferences, different tastes and a different level of requirements. You need to create and follow your own road map to start the journey along your chosen route. The relevant details of our story should simply serve as a comparative 'blue print' on which to model your own chosen route.

Let me give you a brief description of the route my wife and I took to change from the way we were eating that made us fat to the way we reduced our weight. It is a lesson we have had to learn and one that you can simply observe and relate to your own situation.

Before 2002, before we became aware of the true facts of nutrition and the actual facts surrounding the official "healthy eating" advice, we did what most people we knew did. We tried to cut down on the consumption of saturated animal fat and used olive oil or sunflower oil, and the like, for cooking.

We also increased our consumption of carbohydrates, such as, potatoes, beans, pasta, rice, fruit and vegetables. This was easy because we both like these foods very much. In addition, I am very fond of bread, scones, buns and cakes. We were both very happy to follow the official advice for decades even though our weight was slowly creeping up. But something did not add up. Very slowly the question began to be formed in the back our minds. Why did following the "healthy eating" advice produce the result of weight gain instead of the promised weight loss? How could reducing our consumption of fat make us fatter?

My wife was a housewife for a considerable period of our early married life and she liked cooking and preparing the kind of foods that we both wanted to eat. This was common ground between us. However, the way each of us was eating differed slightly.

At home, she was in charge of what we consumed and her guidelines were based on the commonly accepted dogma of 'calories in versus calories out'. In a word, she was keen on counting calories when she decided on the menu for the day. For her, this inevitably meant following one or another popular dieting regime in vogue at any given time. She was nearly always on a diet. To help herself along the way, she had decided not to have breakfast as a normal routine. She usually ended up having a sandwich for lunch and a cooked meal in the evening.

I, on the other hand, travelled a lot in connection with my profession, eating on board ships, in hotels, restaurants, pubs or 'on the go'. I had bread with almost every meal, adored an 'Indian' curry with rice, washed down with a pint or sparkling wine. Chocolate and pudding was always a favourite choice of mine. I have always enjoyed eating and had breakfast, lunch and dinner most days. I also had snacks every day, simply because a couple hours after my meal was swallowed I felt very hungry. This situation was aggravated by the fact that we yo-yoed in and out of any dieting programme we could lay our hands on.

On days when I was with my wife in the office of our small video production company, I started to look at my watch at about 11.30 am to find out if it was lunchtime yet. My wife kept saying: "You can't be hungry yet, you've only just had breakfast!" This was a daily event. I ended up feeling hungry often and had frequent attacks of heart-burn.

The other element of the officially recommended approach to weight control centres on physical exercise.

My wife is not at all keen on exercise for exercise's sake but she did take exercise regularly. For my part, I am a keen tennis player with a background in gymnastics. At every chance that came my way, I played tennis. Sometime I played 2-3 times a week, most often two hours at a time.

As we were following religiously the "healthy eating" advice by cutting down on saturated fat, using polyunsaturated plant based fat and relying on complex carbohydrates for our energy supply while exercising as much as we could, we expected to have the promised rewards as far as our weight was concerned. The outcome should have been that we either reached our normal weight or, at the very least, stopped putting on additional weight.

But neither of us enjoyed the expected result. Following all the advice in terms of food ingredients, counting calories and exercising regularly, my wife simply found that she had fluctuating weight readings on the scales which she used every day. My case was much worse. I put weight on at a steady, seemingly, unstoppable rate. I reached well over 14 stones with a Body Mass Index of over 30, and I should have been 11 stones 2 pounds according to the tables we consulted. Or, as I often said to my friends, I was three inches too short for my weight!

So far, this was the typical situation, repeated in many households up and down the country. By all accounts, this is still the picture in households where obesity is in evidence. It is possible that you recognise this situation yourself.

It is quite on the cards that you, like many an overweight person, have developed a 'sweet tooth' as we did. Do not blame yourself for it. Have a look at the facts behind the love of sugar and sweet things. *This* is one aspect of weight gain *that* cannot be blamed on the official 'healthy eating' advice.

Most mothers start breastfeeding their babies from the moment they are born. It is a natural process. Mothers' milk contains all the nutrients a baby needs to grow and prosper, among them saturated animal fat and a form of sugar - lactose. It also contains enzymes, trace elements and vitamins that protect the baby and aid growth.

What do many mothers do after they stop breastfeeding their babies? They introduce their babies to sweetened processed baby food, sometimes containing high fructose corn syrup. Some even add sugar to the food. The baby takes to the new food and establishes for ever a taste for sweet foods. This is the same whether the baby food in question is made of vegetables, fruit or cereals. Even baby foods that contain meat will also have sugar added to them at the manufacturing stage to enhance the flavour and increase shelf life.

What are most children given as a treat or reward at birthdays or other moments of celebration? Are they given carrots and cheese or are they given sweets, chocolates and cakes? Generations are brought up to associate 'reward' and 'pleasure' with sweet sugary flavours. The result is that it takes a long time for most people to learn to accept other flavours. That is why children learn very slowly to take pleasure in consuming vegetables that introduce a hint of bitter or sour taste. Small babies will grow up to be big adults who retain the same attitude to sweet foods.

Of course, in the days when sweet treats were given to children at birthdays and other times of celebration, these were one day a year indulgences. Now these treats are available daily as part of the load in a shopping trolley.

Now, let's get away from the general observations and return to your own situation. How do you relate to sweet foods, such as cakes, biscuits, ice cream, chocolate and sweetened fizzy drinks? You need to be honest with yourself. A research worker some years ago interviewed a number of overweight people attending a strict weight loss class and asked them what is it that they missed most? The overwhelming majority named the items I have listed above.

Because sugar contains no nutrients and most carbohydrates, such as cereals and refined and manufactured grain products, contain relatively small amounts of nutrients, their consumption simply adds to your energy intake with little or no benefit to you.

As you will see later, cutting down on these foods will provide you with the fastest way of escaping from obesity. Now, let's get on with describing our route map.

Around 2001, a good friend of ours, the husband of a doctor and well versed in health matters, gave us a dieting book to read with the title: *Eat Fat, Get Thin* written by Barry Groves. We had tried every dieting idea, so we read this book too, despite the fact that the title was totally in opposition to the official advice we had so diligently followed.

It was a very disturbing book because Dr. Groves systematically demolished the validity of all the official recommendations. The content of the book seemed well researched and, as such, managed to confuse us unbelievably. We decided to do some research of our own to find out where the truth lay, our motto being never to rely on only one source of information.

The biggest issue for us was the cholesterol question as it seemed to be the corner stone of the official diet advice during the previous 30 years.

It took a little time, but it became evident that the "healthy eating" gospel may have been based on the phoney war on cholesterol initiated by the aforesaid American doctors Gofman and Keys in the early 1950s.

Many scientific reports since that time have proved that the war on consumed cholesterol and everything that followed from it is baseless scientifically and actually causes the unwanted outcomes which it was meant to avoid. The evidence to support Dr. Groves' observations was convincing. But we needed to know more *(see later scientific/historic background)*.

Having read *Eat Fat, Get Thin*, we decided to research four subjects very thoroughly before making changes to our normal way of eating.

First, we needed to know more about the critical issue of cholesterol, because this was the subject that prompted all the other main changes to the eating habits of the population in the USA and in Great Britain and increasingly round the globe, because of its association as a risk factor in heart disease.

Secondly, we wanted to know why the primary sources of human nutrition for millions of years (that is, saturated animal fat, meat, eggs, milk, cream and cheese) suddenly became bad for us in 1953.

Thirdly, we wanted to know what consuming the recommended starches, complex carbohydrates, does to our metabolism?

Finally, we wanted to know what consuming plant based manufactured, polyunsaturated fats, does to our metabolism.

It took us nearly a year to wade through conflicting scientific reports and through epidemiological findings. If you are interested in reading the results of our scientific/historic background to these subjects, I shall detail them at the end of the Chapter.

The challenge we faced was to modify our attitude to cholesterol, calorie counting, saturated animal fat, sugar and complex carbohydrates. We wanted to know more before we changed our ways of eating and we contacted Dr Groves to find out how he came to the views he held about nutrition. We learned that both he and his wife had been obese despite trying every dieting method known to man without success. Then they came across a diet for losing weight which recommended the consumption of saturated animal fat as the main source of energy, in place of starchy carbohydrates. They spent the next 30 years on a high fat and very low carbohydrate diet. Dr Groves has spent that same 30 year period researching the subject of nutrition. During that time both Dr Groves and his wife maintained their normal weight whilst enjoying all their meals.

After we met Dr Groves and his wife, we became convinced that we could do worse than to try out his recommended version of weight control, now supported by our own research findings. It was a very strange experience to begin with as Barry was telling us to forget everything we have been told for the past 20-30 years. The main new issues we had to consider were:

1. What is the role of cholesterol – not just consumed cholesterol - in our bodies?

2. Should we stop eating polyunsaturated plant based fats and spreads and stop using them for cooking? Should we return to eating and using saturated fat?

3. Should or shouldn't we stop counting calories on the basis that this is an inexact practice unless we know the calorific values required for our metabolic processes and for our physical activities at any given moment?

4. Should we cut down on the use of sugar as it is simply supplying calories without any nutritional value?

5. Should we reduce the consumption of refined carbohydrates in our daily meals?

Let's look at each of these issues and our critical findings about them. In this context, some of the information touched upon earlier will, inevitably, be repeated. But, just as we had to be convinced about their validity, you will also need to be convinced in order to proceed along your route with confidence. It is not easy, given the unceasing flow of misinformation given to us daily during the past three to four decades.

1. **Cholesterol:** Cholesterol is a vital substance in the body. It forms the membranes of our cells and constitutes vital bile salts, besides being a precursor of a number of hormones critical to our health. Without cholesterol, no new cells could be formed in our body. If we suffer a bodily injury extra cholesterol is produced to ensure the building of new cells and the healing of the injury. That is what happens when the arteries are injured and inflamed. The cholesterol is accumulating at the point of inflammation in the artery walls to assist the healing process. It is not the cause of Coronary Heart Disease. It is the toxins, the chemical residues

in manufactured food, such as in margarine, and alien foods, such as refined starches, that create the original injury and which are, together, the cause. Cholesterol is simply delivered to the inflamed tissue. This is the view of surgeons, amongst others, after performing many thousands of open heart surgeries.

The liver produces about 80-85% of the cholesterol circulating in the body in a highly controlled manner to supply our daily requirements of this substance. If we consume some cholesterol in our food, the liver simply produces less. However little or however much cholesterol we consume, the liver will adjust accordingly. The final serum cholesterol level will not change significantly.

2. **Saturated Animal Fat:** Research has confirmed that saturated animal fat is stable and contains a number of essential fatty acids among them Omega 3 and Omega 6 in the correct proportions. Without the presence of fatty acids the absorption of vitamins cannot take place. For example, when skimmed milk with added vitamins is consumed, the added vitamins are likely to simply pass through the body without being absorbed because the fat necessary for absorption has been removed. Nature really does know best!

Saturated fat remains stable when heated. This fat was a main ingredient in the traditional foods that humanity consumed for millions of years. The main food sources are: meat, eggs, full fat milk, cream and cheese. It is found in mothers' milk as the most important food ingredient to support growth and healthy development of human babies. Our own metabolism creates saturated animal fat when it stores energy for future use. Our own brain is partly composed of saturated fat.

In contrast, plant based polyunsaturated fats contain linoleic acid in very large quantities, leading to health issues. Polyunsaturated fats are unstable when heated; their molecular structure breaks up and forms various substances, among them trans-fats which are implicated in the development of cancer. Their spreadable versions contain chemical residues from manufacturing processes which are alien to the human metabolism and are harmful to human health.

Prior to the time when agricultural activity started (around 3000 – 5000 years ago), polyunsaturated fats were almost non-existent in the list of foods for human consumption. Since then, grains, seeds, roots and nuts, containing polyunsaturated fat have been gradually introduced as a food ingredient for human consumption. Now they are the officially recommended fats for human consumption.

3. **Calories - to count or not to count:** The basic principle about calories, as far as weight control is concerned, is that if you consume foods that contain the number of calories you need to provide energy for your metabolic processes and for your physical activities, then, your weight will remain stable.

If you consume more calories than you require for your metabolic processes and for providing energy for your physical activities, then your body will store the excess energy in the form of body fat and you will put weight on.

If you consume fewer calories than you require for your metabolic processes and for your physical activities, then you will lose weight because your body will burn up some of your stored fat to make up the difference. There lies the open secret of losing weight!

Having said all that, counting calories, as such, is a futile activity because not all food ingredients that you consume will play a part in the energy equation. Nor do calories from fats, proteins and carbohydrates have the same impact on your metabolic processes.

For example, calories contained in a piece of steak will have a much smaller impact on your weight than a bowl of cereal of the same calorie value, primarily because the protein content of the meat will be largely metabolised as amino acids and will be used for cell building. Whereas the calories contained in cereals and sugar will be used 100% as sources of energy.

One other point emerged regarding calorie counting. Everyone knows that fats contain twice the calories of proteins or carbohydrates. As a consequence, some take the view that the obvious thing to do is to cut down on fat consumption before anything else. But, a little bit like the 'flat earth' hypothesis, this view is based on a false assumption. The important points to remember are these:

- the calories of proteins do not normally form part of the energy exchange;

- the calories contained in consumed carbohydrates, will be part of the energy equation 100% and, if they are surplus to requirements, that energy will be stored as body fat;

- the calories contained in fat, if they are surplus to requirements, will be disseminated in body heat or pass through the body because there would not be any metabolisation of glucose and the consequent insulin activity.

In any case, no-one has a clue how many calories they need at any given moment. But my wife thought that counting calories was the way to see how we were doing, so we continued counting calories.

4. **Sugar:** Sugar is a great favourite ingredient for children and adults alike. The sweet flavour is introduced to the baby in mothers' milk and then continues to be enjoyed by young children who will eat any food with greater enthusiasm if it tastes sweet. Then, grandparents and friends bring chocolates and cakes on every celebratory occasion and none. As adults, many of us who are overweight prefer to drink tea and coffee with a spoonful of sugar, or two. Cakes, biscuits and desserts are considered regular treats.

Fruits contain a form of sugar called fructose. Consumed in fruit, the volume is minimal and is accompanied by fibre which assists in metabolising the fructose. In fruit juice form, the fructose is highly concentrated. In most cases, the fruit juice has added high fructose corn syrup that increases the volume of sugar. This applies equally to fizzy drinks.

Unfortunately, sugar contains no nutrients. It is nothing but empty calories. We now consume as much sugar per week as our great grandparents consumed in a year. Sugar is an alien substance to our metabolic processes and a trigger to a number of modern diseases, not to mention obesity.

5. **Carbohydrates:** Carbohydrates, starchy foods, are the preferred sources of energy according to the 'healthy eating' advice. Consumed mainly in the form of bread, breakfast cereals, biscuits, cakes, pasta, pizza, potatoes, beans, rice and fruit. Besides providing energy, some are providing second class proteins and fibre or roughage. Unfortunately, the manufactured, refined food varieties made up of carbohydrates also contain vegetable-based fat, sugar and salt in large quantities whilst the fibre is mostly removed to allow freezing and increase shelf life.

All these starchy foods end up in the bloodstream as glucose, exactly the same as sugar. As such, they are contributors to the process of putting weight on.

Following the establishment of these facts in our minds, it was a no- brainer. We decided to examine what we were doing right and what we were doing wrong in the light of the nutritional facts we had acquired, with the assistance of Dr Barry Groves, in our research.

That period of reflexion led to two critical developments. First we decided to produce a video programme with Dr Barry Groves. It was called: *Be Slim Without Dieting.*

Secondly, my wife and I started to create a new eating plan to follow in the light of our new knowledge of food ingredients and nutritional requirements.

If you are interested in the historic/scientific background to the above here it is:

Cholesterol is a white waxy material that exists in the body mainly as membranes of the body's cells, especially the nerve cells. It is the raw material that is used for making a range of important substances, such as sex hormones, the hormone cortisol from the adrenal gland, vitamin D, and bile salts. Almost all the cholesterol circulating in the body is synthesized internally by the liver although most cells can produce it if necessary. (Hence the nonsense about the use of Statins.)

Some cholesterol is held in a complex form in solution in the blood combined with lipoprotein. This appears mainly in two combinations, low density lipoprotein (LDL), and high density lipoprotein (HDL). These facilitate the cholesterol being transported in the blood stream. LDL transports newly synthesised cholesterol and triglyceride from the liver to cells where they are needed. HDL collects the cholesterol from dying cells and transports it back to the liver or deposits it in the intestines for excretion if it is not needed to maintain the required level of serum cholesterol.

There is a vacuous scientific view in some quarters that LDL cholesterol is bad and the HDL cholesterol is good! (That is like saying that the ambulance that takes the paramedic to the scene of injury is bad but the ambulance that takes him back to the hospital is good! Author).

So, there is no LDL cholesterol, nor HDL cholesterol. Both LDL and HDL are lipoproteins. There are also other lipoproteins involved in the transportation of cholesterol and triglycerides in the blood stream. These are Chylomicrons and Very Low Density Lipoproteins (VLDL), which are mainly concerned with the transportation of consumed cholesterol from food. There is one called Lp(a) which no-one ever mentions but it is a form of LDL. Inexplicably, they are not normally included in any measurements of the serum cholesterol level.

Nothing shows better the falseness of the science behind the good/bad cholesterol hypothesis and the war on dietary cholesterol than the fact that dietary cholesterol is mainly transported in the blood stream by Chylomicrons or VLDL and not either LDL or HDL.

In terms of size, Chylomicrons are the largest lipoproteins, followed by VLDL, LDL and HDL (the smallest). Each lipoprotein, after delivering the cholesterol and any triglycerides, collapses into the next smaller size and density.

Regarding the causal effects on Coronary Heart Disease, Dr. Dwight Lundell, a heart surgeon of 25 years' experience, carrying out over 5000 open heart surgeries, describes – in an article available on the Internet - the processes involved in the development of this disease in the arteries. He is convinced that it is the inflammation of the artery walls, as the body's natural defence against the invasion of foreign matter (such as, bacteria, toxins, chemical residues in processed food ingredients and viruses) that is the real precursor of Coronary Heart Disease.

As far as food consumption is concerned, the foreign invaders are the toxins and the extensive and continual consumption of foods that our bodies are not used to, such as simple, highly processed carbohydrates and the vegetable oils containing excessive amounts of Omega 6. These cause chronic inflammation and injury in the artery walls that can trap cholesterol which would otherwise freely flow in the bloodstream transported by lipoproteins. In his view, The Diet/Heart hypothesis is fundamentally flawed by blaming dietary cholesterol as the cause for the build-up of plaques under the Endothelium. (arterial wall).

Comparing the constituent elements of butter – a popular source of saturated fat - and a popular margarine available today provides the object lesson for anyone who is interested in their own health.

BUTTER contains milk fat and sometimes a little salt.

A widely consumed margarine (which is the hydrogenated spreadable version of vegetable oils) may contain most or all of the following substances:

- edible oils,
- edible fats,
- salt,
- potassium chloride,
- ascorbil palmitate,
- butylated hydroxyanisole,
- phospholipids,
- tert-butylhydroquinone,
- mono – and di-glycerides of fat forming fatty acids,
- disodium guanylate,
- diacetyltartaric and fatty acid esters of glycerol,

- Propyl octyl or dodecyl gallate,
- tocopherols,
- propylene glycol mono- and di-esters
- sucrose esters of fatty acids,
- curcumin,
- annatto extracts,
- tartaric acids,
- 3,5, trimethylhexenal,
- B-apo-carotenoic acid methyl or ethyl ester,
- skimmed milk powder,
- Xanthopylls,
- Canthaxanthin, and Vitamins A and D.

In view of the findings of Dr Dwight Lundell after 5000 open heart surgeries, the above data underlines his conclusions.

The name Carbohydrates implies that their chemical structure is made up of carbon and water. However, they do not normally contain water; instead they contain hydrogen and oxygen in the same proportion as water. i.e. H_2O.

From the point of view of human consumption, there are two types, unavailable and available. Unavailable carbohydrates are not digestible and they go through the body. We refer to them as fibre in food. However, fibre is none-the-less an important food component because it helps to maintain a healthy gut. (Vegetables, especially green vegetables, and fresh fruit will supply plenty of fibre.)

Available carbohydrates consist of monosaccharides. Two monosaccharides can join together to form a disaccharide. The commonest monosaccharides are glucose, fructose and galactose. The three best known disaccharides are a) sucrose – the common sugar – which is composed of glucose joined to fructose; b) lactose, found in milk, which is composed of glucose joined to galactose; and c) maltose which consists of two glucose units joined together.

Carbohydrates are nothing more or less than a complex mixture of sugars. They simply provide energy in a diet with little or no nutrients. It defies logic to warn against the consumption of sugar but recommend the consumption of carbohydrates. They all end up as glucose in the bloodstream. (Consumed in the form of bread, for example, they can also provide some protein and dietary fibre.)

Dr. George V Mann, participant in the Framingham Study, the largest continuing research into the subject, and researcher of the African Masai tribe wrote:

"The diet/heart hypothesis has been repeatedly shown to be wrong, and yet, for complicated reasons of pride, profit and prejudice, the hypothesis continues to be exploited by scientists, fund-raising enterprises, food companies and even government agencies. The public is being deceived by the greatest health scam of the century"

Much more information is available on:
www.pubmed.org
www.thincs.org
www.second-opinions.co.uk
www.drpeeke.com

5

Planning the dietary changes

When we set out to modify our normal way of eating in order to regain our desired weight, we did not have the benefit of the necessary scientific and nutritional knowledge that is available today. That was why we spent so much time and effort finding out as much as we could about food. Unfortunately, the relevant facts were not easily available from health professionals or from dieticians, educated in the orbit of the diet/heart hypothesis during the past 30 years, most of whom would rather give you advice than information.

We started by doing our own Reality Checks. We found that we lived on sugar a great deal of the time, not just the white stuff but also the sugars contained in the scones, biscuits, pizza, breakfast cereals, cakes, chocolate, ice creams and desserts we consumed. Added to this was the sugar contained in the soft drinks we drank, including fruit juice.

We consumed all these sugar sources because we loved to eat these types of food in meals and as snacks. We know now that these are mainly sources of energy and, evidently, we were having too much of these items because we were putting on weight. We consumed too much energy which we did not need despite the counting of calories.

Sometimes we grabbed a readymade meal or two from supermarket shelves, unaware of the fact that they were packed with plant based hydrogenated fats, sugar and salt.

So, given our addiction to sweet things and to lovely bread and scones and chips, we had to look at how we needed to change things, how we needed to reduce the energy we were consuming without feeling hungry.

We then looked at all the other stuff we have regularly eaten. Both my wife and I loved fish in any shape or form, chicken, beef, pork, lamb and duck as our meat sources. We also consumed eggs, cream and cheese. As we realised after our research, these foods provided most of our required nutrients, vitamins, minerals and trace elements, especially as we supplemented these with green vegetables.

There was a savoury dish that posed a major problem which we simply had to face – fish and chips. This meal was a favourite 'takeaway' for us, despite the fact that it contains carbohydrates in the form of batter and potatoes, soaked in polyunsaturated hot oil. We realised that this was a deadly combination.

Then we looked at how we prepared our meals. We noted that we were using either olive oil or sun flower oil for cooking, avoiding the use of saturated animal fat. Now in possession of the facts, we immediately decided to change back to cooking with saturated fat, such as lard, butter and duck fat and, our favourite, goose fat. We continued to use olive oil as it is a monounsaturated fat, stable enough for cooking and dressing meals; and anyway, we like the flavour of olive oil.

We looked at the way we consumed vegetables and fruit, especially the official advice of having five portions of each per day for a healthy life.

We thought that we did OK on that score (although we certainly did not meet the five a day criterion). We liked onions, potatoes, tomatoes, cabbage, broccoli, Brussels sprouts, beans, peas, carrots and spinach and we used them in the right way in our meals.

Fruit was a problem, not because we did not like fruit, but because we did not get round to eating fruit all that often. Generally, we liked apples, pears, grapes, bananas, strawberries and raspberries. Then, the realisation hit. All these items are essentially carbohydrates, adding to the intake of energy. So, they should be considered with the other carbohydrate foods when we decide how we best to change our diet. We realised we would need a list of priorities to follow.

The conclusion we drew after first examination was that we needed to prepare three lists.

- **List 1:** the food ingredients that we would like to keep in our new menus.

- **List 2:** the food ingredients that we may like to have occasionally but which we could give up if we needed to.

- **List 3:** the food ingredients that we must give up either straightaway or gradually in order to achieve the greatest reduction in the intake of calories and start our weight loss.

This all sounds very methodical and orderly. It certainly was not. We argued. We each had our own favourite foods we wanted to keep eating. It took some haggling, checking the relative energy content of food items that we had to discard or wanted to keep. Chocolate was a key issue between us. We compromised by deciding to keep the chocolate but switch from the sugar rich milk chocolate to a darker version with about 70% cocoa content.

In preparation of our first list, we consulted a modern recommendation based on the traditional diet of humanity well before the 'healthy eating' advice was ever mooted.

The traditional food ingredients were made up of meat, fish, eggs, milk, cream, cheese, berries, fruit and nuts. The only method of processing these foods was by simply cooking some of them after fire had been tamed for human use. That was between 50,000 and 100,000 years ago.

The modern recommendation, based on current scientific understanding, places these food ingredients into four groups, based on the nutrients they provide:

- **Group 1:** full fat milk and cheese
- **Group 2:** meat, fish and eggs
- **Group 3:** fruit and vegetables
- **Group 4:** butter and cream

The idea was that one should take foods from each of the four groups twice a day. This should include at least half pint of full fat milk. That would mean that the carbohydrate intake would be reduced to what is available from the milk the vegetables and fruits. This is the best scenario for maximum weight loss but we were doubtful if we could give up some of our other favourite meals made up of carbohydrates such as bread, pasta and potatoes, at least, not entirely.

In preparing the second list my wife and I argued over things like, how often should we have an Indian 'takeaway', in view of the fact that it usually comes with rice. Rice contains a lot of starch. Then we looked at potatoes and bread. We both liked chips, cream potatoes, baked potatoes and crisps. We decided that we should retain baked potatoes and the occasional portion of chips. Bread was another issue. My wife felt it reasonably easy to cut down on her bread consumption, except that she liked to have the occasional slice of toast with marmite and lashings of butter.

One of the most difficult decisions we had to take concerned muesli for breakfast. Why? Because we used to like to have it and because some varieties were made with rolled cereals, such as wheat or rye, rolled oats or cornflakes, in a word, carbohydrates. More desirable varieties are made with rolled or whole grain oats with added nuts and seeds, topped with fresh fruits. Under the name muesli one can have two different breakfasts with completely different nutrients and energy content, with or without added sugar or honey.

In this context, we considered nuts and seeds. Nuts are very good sources of Omega 3 and 6 fatty acids, vitamin E, and trace minerals such as magnesium, selenium, potassium and phosphorus. All of these assist the vital hormone activities in the body. We liked almonds, Brazil nuts, chestnuts and hazel nuts. Peanuts and cashew nuts were also used sometimes, mainly accompanied by a glass or two of you-know-what. We decided to continue enjoying the nuts we have been consuming before, primarily for their nutrient values and the fibre they provide.

We developed a similar attitude to edible seeds. Our favourites were sesame seeds, poppy seeds, sunflower seeds and pumpkin seeds. These are all very good sources of a whole range of vitamins, trace elements, protein and fibre. They can be eaten raw or dried, and can be used in cooking. They were here to stay.

Biscuits and cakes were another issue. We decided to elbow biscuits and most cake consumption, but maintain having lovely scones with clotted cream and jam as an occasional treat.

As far as salad leaves and green vegetables were concerned this was not an issue as they contain minimal starches in relation to other nutrients so can be freely consumed in large quantities. Fruits do contain fructose but as we consume a limited amount of fruit, we could monitor how things would develop in the future. Fruit juice, however, with its fructose concentrate and no fibre benefits, had to go.

In preparing the third list, one thing we agreed immediately. We must cut down severely on our sugar consumption despite our addiction to sugary foods. We made a decision straightaway that first we would cut out sugar in our tea and coffee as soon as possible. It was strange at first but within a week my wife switched to a popular sweetener and I cut out sugar altogether. It was actually fun after a day or two since I discovered the flavours in both tea and coffee that were hidden before by the sweetness of sugar. Within a few weeks my wife gave up sugar substitutes too.

We also stopped drinking colas and other fizzy drinks once we learned that the manufacturers put high fructose corn syrup or 10 to 30 spoonsful of sugar per bottle in them to enhance their impact on our taste buds. These changes alone achieved a cut in our energy intake of hundreds of calories a day.

A curious and unexpected experience resulted from this development. We suddenly found that some of our favourite cakes and puddings tasted too sweet. As a result, we started wanting fewer of them and made them with less sugar and without sugary toppings.

The third list began to write itself really as we began to experience new flavours in place of sweetness. We stopped having cereals for breakfast and switched to boiled eggs or bacon and eggs with only one piece of toast. Eventually we discarded the toast altogether.

The same thing happened to pasta and all other foods made of flour. We decided to cut these down gradually, effectively, having them once a fortnight; later that became once a month. Again, we were rewarded by a new sensation. When we did have these foods they became a treat and we enjoyed them far more than previously.

In order to help our efforts and to avoid any deviation in weaker moments, we also decided that we would not buy anything that we should not eat so as not to have these items in the house at all. Put it another way, the first place to exercise weight control is in your shopping trolley! The money we saved on not buying these body fat-producing items allowed us to buy more valuable, nutritional and interesting foods. The biggest saving was achieved by not buying ready-made foods and sugary cakes and biscuits.

Here I am talking about events that took 4-5 months involving the proverbial trial and error. It was not easy. Old habits die hard. Luckily, we started losing weight right from the start, which helped.

My wife, who was not greatly over her normal weight, began to shed about a pound a week. I, on the other hand, started to lose over two pounds per week. This was an exciting outcome and became the main incentive for doing more along the path of weight reduction. The heavier you are, the greater the weight loss at the start. (The nearer we get to our normal weight the slower the weight loss but by then you should have changed your eating habits for good.)

One other welcome development was the fact that I stopped feeling as hungry as I did before our change of diet. It made sense on two counts:

* first, having reduced the over consumption of sugar and carbohydrates, we had also reduced the insulin clear-out of glucose from the blood and the consequent feeling of hunger

* secondly, the increased consumption of saturated fat meant that food stayed in the digestive system longer due to its relatively slower digestion

Suddenly, as a direct consequence of these developments, I became aware of a new consideration: portion sizes. I became aware of the fact that my eyes required me to put as much food on my plate as it could hold. This visual requirement had developed through a number of years without me being consciously aware of it. As our former eating habits were based on the 'healthy eating' advice and were concentrated on starches, the continuous glucose spikes after each meal triggered the insulin reaction and the clearing out of glucose from my blood, making me hungry soon after eating. My subconscious reaction to this was, apparently, to increase of portion size on my plate in order to avoid feeling hungry so quickly.

With hindsight, this was the worst thing I could have done, as it did not result in the desired effect but simply increased the volume and calories I consumed, resulting in putting weight on. My stomach had grown to accommodate the increased volume of food and my eyes bathed in the welcome sight of a mountain of tasty food on my plate.

Now that our food intake has changed to a more nutritional variety with a reduced glucose creating component, the hunger issue has subsided and the food I used to pile on my plate appeared too much. It was too much. The appetite control in my brain, the appestat, suddenly re-established its function. Both my wife and I gradually reduced the portion size at every meal. Also, we appeared to have cut out the habit of snacking. We did not feel hungry between meals nor did we crave for sweet things any longer. These new developments turned out to be most significant, with a huge impact on our weight control.

During the following months, I lost 20 pounds - that is 1stone and 6 pounds. I was delighted. I became much more active, feeling lighter and more confident and enjoying and discovering the new flavours which were hidden by the sweetness in food.

Very soon we arrived at new menus which we both liked to follow and which still form the basis of our diet eleven years later. My wife is now happy at her normal weight and I am content to be only about 5-6 pounds over my 'ideal' weight because I am a piglet. We no longer stick rigidly to our original lists.

When on holiday or visiting friends we eat what we like. If it means that we put on one or two pounds in a week, as is often the case, we return home and continue with our normal ways of eating. The extra pounds naturally disappear within a few weeks. I can say with a happy smile on my face that we no longer have a weight problem. (My wife disagrees. She thinks I still do!) Nor do we have any of the health issues normally associated with being overweight or obese. On the contrary, our appetite is again controlled by our appestat in the natural way. We now only feel hungry if our next meal is delayed by several hours for one reason or another. It is a good place to be in.

Now there is one issue that can (and did) cause some soul searching. How should we relate to alcohol? We both like to drink wine, mainly with meals preceded by an aperitif or two. The fact is that alcohol behaves exactly as if it was a carbohydrate except that it absorbs and metabolises much quicker. If it is consumed with a meal it is metabolised first. For example, when we had an Indian 'takeaway' with rice and a glass of wine, the calories in the wine took precedence in providing us with energy and the calories in the rice and the rest of the meal would probably end up as body fat.

The answer to the question of alcohol was to treat it as another form of carbohydrate in the new scheme of things. This is another way of saying that we included wine in the first list and decided to halve its consumption immediately and take a final decision on it later (much later). We only drank wine with meals, anyway.

Looking back on the experience, we both agree that it was quite easy to make the necessary changes, despite the fact that, at the beginning, we did not know what we were doing. Also, we were understandably somewhat hesitant in making changes that were in direct opposition to the officially promoted 'healthy eating' advice.

But, the proof of the pudding is in the eating, as they say!

We enjoy one other new development which has nothing to do with weight control. It is the amount of money we save on not buying food that puts weight on us. Although we spend more on fish, meat, eggs, cream and cheese, there is still a small amount of saving on our food bill, not least because the actual amount of food we now eat to satisfy our nutritional needs and hunger is reduced. It is a win, win situation.

To retrace our path, leaving out the trial and error aspects, we have made the following important steps:

1. We created a list of food stuffs that provide the most calories in a meal without providing any or many nutrients. Sugar and sources of refined carbohydrates were the main items here. In particular, cakes, biscuits, jams, honey, flavoured milk shakes, concentrated fruit juices and fizzy drinks were the main targets. We also stopped buying manufactured, processed food.

2. We decided to reduce the use of sugar in tea and coffee, eventually eliminating it altogether. We also stopped drinking alcopops and sugar rich fizzy drinks and reduced the frequency of eating ice-cream.

3. According to what we had learned about nutrition, this plan should already have made a huge impact on our energy input and that is exactly what happened. We started to lose weight within a week.

4. We then looked at the food ingredients that would give us the best sources of saturated fat, having decided to stop using polyunsaturated vegetable oils. We made an exception for olive oil as it is a mono-unsaturated oil which means it is more stable even when heated. We decided to use and consume more full fat milk,

cream, cheese, eggs and fish, lamb, chicken, duck, pork and beef.

5. We also looked at what vegetables we wanted to continue eating. We liked all green vegetables, plus peppers, tomatoes, squash, carrots and aubergines and all of these stayed on our list as sources of relatively low carbohydrate content. We both wanted to continue using potatoes so we kept creamed potatoes, made with butter and milk, and jacket potatoes, but allowed ourselves very few chips.

6. We created a new list of meals and food ingredients showing the level of energy and nutrients they provide. I reproduce this list for you to look at in Appendix 1.

7. We then looked for new recipes for breakfast, lunch and dinner which would allow us to follow the recommendation included in the four Groups of Foods of which we should have two portions per day.

8. Interestingly enough, this process created a new level of interest in food. We both became rather excited in anticipation of the impact these changes would have on our weight. My wife checked her weight every day and continues to do so even today. I weigh myself about once a week to avoid the variations caused by different daily activity patterns.

9. We also noticed that the new and different combinations of food ingredients gave us new flavours to enjoy. We have developed new favourite meals. I shall give you later a list of some of these meals for your consideration.

Critically, there were two practical but simple measures we took at the start of our road plan. First, we looked at the content of our fridge and freezer and cleared out the items we did not wish to consume anymore. The idea was simple enough - if we do not have to hand anything we have been addicted to by way of food ingredients, it is easier to avoid the temptation to have them. Secondly, we realised that the primary control measure we needed to take was right at the shopping trolley in the supermarket. That is to say, if you do not put any of the items in the trolley that you have decided not to eat, then you do not have them at home to tempt you. It is like dealing with any addiction, for example, smoking; if you do not have any cigarettes at home, you cannot smoke.

I learned this lesson when I gave up smoking. Like any addiction, there are a number of components one needs to tackle. In the case of smoking, it was nicotine addiction and a conditioned reflex. Conditioned reflex for me was when, faced by any form of stress, I started to tap all the pockets to see where the cigarettes were. Each time this happened, my method was to think of something which I wanted more than a cigarette. It worked for me. Anyway, back to the measures relating to food.

In the supermarket, before we put anything in the trolley, we started to look at the labels more closely, checking the carbohydrate content of the bag, box or can, particularly the sugar content. Previously, we were only interested in 'sell-by-date' or 'consume-by-date'. It really is amazing what you can find once you are aware of the nutritional values of food. These are the things you can find representing sugar content:

- **Agave syrup** is a commercially produced sweetener. It largely consists of fructose.
- **Concentrated fruit juices** mostly contain fructose in high quantities.
- **Fructose** is, in fact naturally occurring in fruit but now commercially manufactured and used in a variety of processed foods.
- **High fructose corn syrup** is a thick syrup made from the starches of corn or maize. Widely used as a sweetener in manufactured food.
- **Isomalt** is another sugar alcohol used a lot in cake decorations due to its crystal-like appearance.
- **Maltitol** is another sugar alcohol that is used in chocolate, ice-cream and sweets.
- **Mannitol** is another sugar alcohol used in hard sweets.
- **Polydextrose** is different in that it is a synthetic soluble fibre that is used as a sweetener in cereals, cakes and salad dressings.
- **Sorbitol** is a sugar alcohol made from corn syrup.

It is no accident that the population of the developed world is ballooning relentlessly when consuming all those hidden and useless calories totally unaware of doing so.

The practical outcome of all this label gazing was that we started to distinguish between various products of the same kind. For example, we chose shortbread fingers instead of cereal bars; granary wholemeal bread instead of fruit loaves; marmite and peanut butter instead of jams and chocolate spread; pears, kiwi fruit, raspberries and gooseberries instead of pine apples, bananas, oranges, grapes and melons; butter instead of low fat vegetable spreads, full fat milk instead of skimmed or flavoured, semi-skimmed milk – to name a few. The list could go on.

As I said before, you do not need to follow our steps. But, have a look at what we have done. Our steps suited us and set us onto the right path. Of course, you may take exactly the same route but it is more likely that you will diverge here and there to suit your own lifestyle and preferences. You can make all your changes immediately for immediate effect. This is likely to depend on how heavy you are and how much weight you need to lose to ease the discomforts that you have to put up with.

Evidence is out there that weight loss can result in reduced symptoms of type 2 diabetes, high blood pressure and asthma, not to mention the pressure on the joints. There are no evident health issues that would not benefit from reducing your weight if you are overweight. However, all health issues relating to weight loss should be discussed with your health professionals.

The only advice I would like to give is to keep going along the path you have chosen, modifying it as you go along, based on the results you achieve. You will succeed if you do that and life will begin anew.

In parallel with changing the food we used to eat to a more nutritious variety, we became aware of another important consideration – portion sizes. It is a well-known saying that you are eating with your eyes. A plate filled to the brim with delicious food is a very satisfying sight. It is easy to get into the habit of piling food onto a plate until there is a danger that some will fall off. This becomes a habit -

a very bad one. Meals rich in carbohydrates do not trigger the natural appetite controlling signal and this allows us to over eat without control.

But soon after we switched to more nutritious meals, we began to notice that what we put on our plates proved to be too much. Consequently, a gradual reduction of the portions we consumed accelerated the weight loss we experienced. A very good lesson to be learned along the way of escaping from obesity!

From our own experience it is clear that making the change from the way of eating which made you obese to the new plan must be made at a speed to suit you. The most important change is likely to be the escape from an addiction to sweet tasting foods. Sugar is a deadly substance and it controls most people's eating habits. Going 'cold turkey' often does not work and, anyway, there is no need for such a sudden and brutal change.

It is more important to make your changes permanent rather than fast. The lesson is to start with sugar itself, then eliminate the other sweet things one by one. Once you have dealt with sugar, the carbohydrate component in meals can be addressed. Remember, as far as your digestive system is concerned, all carbohydrates turn into glucose – or blood sugar – just like sugar does.

To succeed, clearly one must keep going and the results will please you and encourage you. Our experience was that it gets easier as time goes by because you will start enjoying other flavours and feel better, feel more energetic and feel less joint pain.

6

Our chosen ingredients

The most interesting period in our quest to get back to our normal weight was when we started experimenting with our chosen food ingredients. We would like to share this experience with you because we hope that the content of this chapter will catch your imagination and will give you as much pleasure as it did us. I will group our chosen ingredients into six groups:

* Meats
* Fish
* Eggs
* Dairy products
* Vegetables
* Fruits

Meats

Let's start with meats. We have chosen poultry (such as chicken, turkey, duck and goose) and beef, lamb, pork and venison.

- **Chicken** is a most popular meat product, cheap and widely available. Most people think about chicken as breast of chicken. We do not like breast of chicken because it is the driest piece of the bird providing the least flavour. But, for some inexplicable reason – may be herd instinct – most people buy it and most restaurants serve it. It is also the most expensive portion to buy.

  We prefer a leg of chicken, particularly thigh. Both the 'drum stick', and thigh are more tasty and moist than the breast. Also, the skin on these can be cooked to be crisp and crackly. Most of all, the leg is less expensive than the breast meat. Inexplicable!

  One of the most favourite ways we eat chicken thighs is baked over a layer of sliced potatoes and slices of chorizo, a Spanish sausage. We usually serve with it some steamed broccoli, or other green vegetables.

  Another way of serving chicken thighs is to prepare a paprika stew with fried onions, garlic, chopped peppers and tomatoes and cook the meat in this sauce until tender. It is a Hungarian favourite. We serve this topped with soured cream, with creamed potatoes and cucumber salad. Superb!

  Sometimes, we buy a tray of chicken legs – very cheap – and make a large saucepan of chicken soup which we can consume for several days, or freeze some of it for later use.

Another treat is to dip the thighs in seasoned flour, beaten eggs and bread crumbs, before frying them in duck or goose fat; a great meal with a green salad.

We came across a great find when it comes to flavour - smoked chicken. Strips of smoked chicken stir fried in duck fat with onions, peppers, garlic, tomatoes make super meal which is easily prepared. It can be eaten hot, or used as sandwich filling to take to the office. Thigh or drum stick with a salad also serves as a good packed lunch.

* **Turkey** is a popular choice for most people at Christmas. We have chosen to ignore turkey at Christmas and have it only as an occasional meal. Again, probably for the same reason, we choose to buy a leg of turkey. One leg, roasted under foil then browned will give us at least two meals and is delicious served with red cabbage, wilted in goose fat and seasoned.

* **Duck** is also a favourite with us. Either we buy a whole duck for roasting or just the breast. We fry the breast skin side down in a frying pan, and then when the skin is nice and brown, bake it in the oven under foil. We can serve this in a variety of ways, depending on how we feel.

* **Goose** has become our all-time favourite at Christmas. Although it is an expensive bird, it has the one great benefit of providing bowls of delicious goose fat for cooking and making the most wonderful roast potatoes. In our view, it is the most flavoursome of poultry. Practically all the bird can be used in meals.

When the last morsel of meat has been enjoyed, use the carcass, boiled with herbs and onions, to produce a wonderful stock for future use.

* **Red meats -** our favourites are beef, lamb, pork and veal, and we experimented with venison and ostrich.

* **Beef -** the most popular cuts are fillet, sirloin and rump steaks. These cuts are widely used as grilled steaks or roast beef. They are all rather expensive cuts. We like them all but actually prefer a piece of beef cut from a fore rib. One of the best ways to prepare a steak for flavour is on the BBQ.

Of course, the most popular way to eat beef is to roast it. It is our favourite too. This is the time when roast potatoes are a must with lots of rich gravy. What the hell! You do not have it every day. Unless you cannot bear to do without it, it is best to sacrifice the Yorkshire pudding and add extra vegetables instead.

We have found that if you buy the cheapest cut with a reputation of being quiet tough and cook it very slowly on a low temperature, then barbeque it, the toughness vanishes and it will be tender and flavoursome. This applies to the cheaper cuts of beef, such as, brisket.

A new way of cooking any tougher cuts of meat is under vacuum, or *sous vide*, as the French say. You need to invest a few quid before you can do this. You require a special water bath with an accurate temperature control. You also need a vacuum sealing machine and a roll of suitable plastic bags. The chosen meat is placed in the bag and vacuum sealed. The water oven is set at a particular temperature, depending on whether you wish to eat the meat rare, medium rare, medium or well done. The entire piece of meat will be cooked at this set temperature in a number of hours.

Our chosen setting for beef is 55C for 8 hours or more. You can leave it in the water as long as you like as it will not overcook. Just before you are ready to serve, remove the meat from the vacuum bag and either BBQ it, pop it into a very hot oven, or seal it all round in a hot frying pan. A wonderfully tender and flavoursome piece of meat will be on your plate.

- **Lamb -** we buy a leg of lamb or shoulder for roasting or lamb chops or cutlets for grilling. Occasionally we buy lamb knuckle for braising which makes a good warm winter meal, as does a best end of neck for 'hot pot'.

- **Pork -** we have indulged in a great deal of experimentation with pork. We like pork in many different forms. Bacon, pork belly, chops, shoulder, are the favoured cuts. I even like trotters in aspic but my wife is less keen. We have some of our recipes detailed later on.

Fish

We never had any trouble deciding what to do with fish in our new approach to food. We both love fish as well as shellfish. Having lived in Whitstable, on the North Kent Coast, we never had a problem getting a huge selection of fresh fish. We love smoked salmon, although it is a pricey food. Smoked trout or kippers are less expensive and equally flavoursome. Haddock cooked in milk is a favourite with us. We often had crabs and prawns and, occasionally, lobster. Prawns, cooked in garlic butter, stands out as a treat. Brown crab meat can be used in a variety of ways. For example, it can be mixed with cream to fill ravioli. Fish, like salmon and trout, is a rich source of omega 3 fatty acid. Other fish, including crayfish, are very good sources of high quality proteins, that is, essential amino acids and iodine. Fish oil is also a natural source of Vitamin D.

One fish dish we do have a problem with is fish and chips, normally cod and chips. Not because we did not like cod but because the batter, the vegetable oil it was fried in, and the chips with it, are the worst combination of food when you are trying to lose weight.

Eggs

We normally think of chicken eggs when we talk about eggs because we eat them in vast quantities and in so many ways. Chefs sometimes use quails' eggs and duck eggs. We do not have experience in consuming anything other than goose eggs and chicken eggs and an occasional quails' egg in restaurants. Be that as it may, eggs are very important sources of nutrients.

In the 1950-60s by far the best public advice was aired on British television: "Go to work on an egg". All those of a certain age will remember this. It not only implied that one should have a good breakfast in the morning, but also recommended a most nutritional breakfast ingredient.

Let me remind you that an egg creates and supports life. All of its content is there to do this job. You might be surprised to see how much just one little egg will give you.

Energy	277/66kJ/kcal
Protein	6.4g
Carbohydrate	trace
Fat	4.6g
Saturated fatty acids	1.3g
Monounsaturated f.a	1.7g
Polyunsaturated f.a.	0.7g
n-3 PUFA	0.07g
of which DHA	0.03g
n-6 PUFA	0.66g
Cholesterol	177mg
Dietary fibre	none
Minerals and Trace Elements	
Sodium	78mg
Potassium	73mg
Calcium	23mg
Phosphorus	91mg
Magnesium	7mg
Chloride	91mg
Iron	0.9mg
Zinc	0.6mg
Copper	0.03mg
Iodine	25µg
Selenium	12µg
Vitamins	
Vitamin A	64µg
Vitamin D	1.6µg
Vitamin E	0.7mg
Vitamin K2	3.5µg
Vitamin C	none
Thiamin (vitamin B1)	0.04mg
Riboflavin (vitamin B2)	0.25mg
Niacin	0.03mg
Vitamin B6	0.07mg
Folate	24µg

Vitamin B12	1.4µg
Biotin	10µg
Pantothenic Acid	0.7mg
Choline	144mg

Isn't that amazing?

It is now almost impossible to believe that, because of the sudden appearance of the dubious Diet/Heart hypothesis, the "Go to work on an egg" advice was not only discontinued but it was replaced with a warning not to have more than one egg a week. And why was that, you may ask? Because of the cholesterol content, of course. Nothing illustrates more eloquently the senseless phoney war on cholesterol than this change in public recommendation by those whose job it is supposed to be to safeguard public health.

We love eggs and eat them every day. We have created a variety of recipes for preparing eggs for breakfast as well as for other meals. I will list these recipes later.

Milk Products

- **Cow's milk -** When we first started out on our journey to get to our normal weight, we had to refocus on milk. As was recommended to the public, we used skimmed milk with added vitamins in teas and coffees and for cooking. We did not like the taste of it and it took some getting used to but we were told that it was healthier, so we persevered. We were quite angry when we learned that it was useless to have added vitamins in a product if there are no fatty acids present; the vitamins cannot be absorbed and simply pass through the body. In actual fact the added vitamins were simply a marketing ploy. Later, we found out that, during the production of skimmed milk, whitening chemicals are added to it – the same substance that is added to brilliant white industrial paint – because skimmed milk has a bluish grey natural colour without it and, as such, is not very appealing to the eye.

We switched to milk and milk products in stages. First, we switched to full fat milk. The flavour and its creamy texture, in comparison to skimmed milk, was a source of long forgotten delights.

* **Cream –** Our investigation into milk led almost immediately to our taking a new look at creams. We did use cream previously but, again, single cream, soured cream and, on occasions, whipping cream.

Now the horizon has opened up embracing double cream and clotted cream. New ways to use them developed. My wife is a good cook and this development gave her renewed interest in experimenting with new flavours and textures.

* **Cheese -** We always liked cheese. My wife loves Cheddar in particular in all shapes and forms, saying that it is so versatile. So do I, but I prefer Stilton. By way of experimenting, we decided to branch out and sampled some French varieties, in particular, Reblochon, Compte and Epoisse. We also came across some goat's and sheep's cheese. These we have found a little strange at first because of flavours that require a little time to get used to. We did in the end. We are still experimenting.

A whole new world of flavours entered our pallets experimenting with cheese while, at the same time, the nutritional content of our meals improved.

Vegetables

Basically, we learned to classify our favoured vegetables into two groups: those which contain less starch and are safe to eat in any quantities and those which are high in carbohydrate and have high glycaemic index to be consumed with care.

The first group of vegetables included: Brussels sprouts, broccoli, garlic, cucumber, peas, tomatoes, peppers, fennel, cabbage, radishes and lettuce. The second group included potatoes, squash, onions, beans, carrots, sweetcorn and parsnips.

* **Potatoes** - Thinking back to the time when we started to change our attitude to food, vegetables caused quite a problem. The reason for this was the conflict between our awareness of their carbohydrate content of some of the favourites. Potatoes were the biggest issue. We both love potatoes in all forms.

  Chips are the biggest problem because they combine two sources of energy in one mouthful; starches and fat. Why is that a problem? Because of the three primary sources of nutrients, carbohydrates, proteins and fat, only carbohydrates and fats are used in the energy exchange that is the consumption and use of energy. Proteins are not normally involved. As chips contain both carbohydrates and fat, eating them means that carbohydrates metabolise immediately into glucose and the fat continues to metabolise but at a *slower* rate. It is unlikely that all the carbohydrate calories consumed in one go will be used up before an insulin dump into the blood stream will clear it of glucose and deposit it as body fat.

Another favourite of ours is creamed potatoes. This food has the same problem as chips; starches and fat combined, due to the fact that we make it with plenty of butter. (This is a treat for rare occasions only!)

The third way we like to prepare potatoes is baked in the oven, served with lashings of butter or soured cream. You cannot get away from the fact that, whichever method is used, a combination of starches and fat is likely to happen. So, we decided not to exclude potatoes from our new regime but to cut our consumption down. In that regard, we learned that we could substitute potatoes with Butternut Squash. Boiled and mashed with a little butter is not at all bad.

- **Onions, peppers and garlic** –These versatile vegetables can be_ eaten raw and they can be used as cooking ingredients. (Garlic may be an exception to 'eating raw'.) Many dishes start with frying chopped onions, with or without garlic, in preparation for soups and stews, not to mention savoury pies. One of my favourite chicken recipes starts with frying all three of them and adding tomatoes and paprika spice. All of these contain lower levels of starches and sugars than potatoes.

- **Peas, beans, carrots, sweetcorn, cabbage, Brussels sprouts, broccoli, fennel, parsnips** - Vegetables like these are mainly used to accompany a meat or a fish dish. They can all be cooked in water but they are even nicer when steamed and retain some of their firmness. Parsnips are the ones with the highest content of starches with a high glycaemic index.

* **Cucumber, radishes and lettuce** - A great variety of salads can be created from these vegetables. They can be combined with peppers and tomatoes from the list above. One of my favourite cucumber salads is made by thinly slicing the cucumber, laying the slices down on a large plate, sprinkling them with salt. After about one hour, squeeze the salty liquid out and place the meat of the cucumber into a mixture of water, sugar and vinegar (to taste) and leave to rest in a fridge for another hour. Sprinkle with ground black pepper or cayenne pepper and serve as an accompaniment to the main meal.

As we are on to recipes, I will provide some of our most favourite recipes for breakfast, lunch and dinner in the next chapter. For those who are new to cooking, I also describe the method of preparation we followed.

Fruits

We spent a lot of time looking at fruit during our deliberations. There were two reasons for this. First, we like most types of fruit; secondly, some have had a bad reputation due to their relatively high fructose content. What we actually learned about fruit was an absolute eye opener. Fruits are important food ingredients, so I give you chapter and verse of our findings.

Fruits are, in general, not only delicious to eat but they also provide us with a whole range of antioxidants in the form of vitamins, minerals and phytochemicals to protect our bodies against the harmful effects of free radicals. Fruit is also a good source of soluble fibre which slows down digestion and delays the emptying of the stomach, making us feel full for longer.

Ideally, we always tried to buy fresh fruit when we could, but, of course there is more to it than meets the eye. Picking and eating fruit, ripe and fresh from the tree, is a romantic notion which, sadly for most us, is far from reality. But do not think of frozen fruit as the poor relation of its fresh counterpart. As soon as fruit is harvested it starts to lose its nutrients and significant losses can occur between orchard and plate. Frozen fruit is processed immediately after picking, thereby locking all its nutrients in place until defrosted and eaten; this also applies to frozen vegetables.

This is what we have found most revealing about the fruits we love to eat.

* **Apples** - among the most common of all fruits and there is a wide variety of them. They are high in antioxidants, most of which are found in the peel so don't be tempted to discard this. They also benefit our health by lessening the absorption of glucose, stimulating pancreatic cells to secrete insulin and increasing the uptake of glucose from the blood by stimulating insulin receptors. Apples are also believed to have a number of properties that could help reduce the risk of cancer, including anti-mutagenic and anti-inflammatory mechanisms. Small wonder that it has

long been believed by previous generations that 'an apple a day keeps the doctor away'.

* **Avocados** - a nutritional power house with numerous potential health benefits. They are rich in oleic acid, a monounsaturated fat and contain around 4 grams of protein, far more than most other fruits. In addition they are an excellent source of Vitamins K, B9, 6 and 5, C & E.

* **Bananas** - perfectly packaged to fit into a weight loss plan. Being highly portable and naturally sweet, they can help curb any mid-afternoon sugar cravings at a quarter of the calories you would find in a chocolate bar. Additionally about half of its fibre is soluble, leaving you feeling fuller for longer. As well as containing the essential B group vitamins, including the highest amount of B6 in any fruit, bananas are an excellent source of the essential mineral, potassium which helps to regulate blood pressure and maintain proper heart function. Rich in pectin, bananas aid digestion and stimulate the growth of friendly bacteria in the bowel as well as producing digestive enzymes to assist in the absorption of nutrients, whilst, being a natural antacid, they provide relief from acid reflux and heartburn.

* **Berries** - rich in antioxidants but it is the Blueberry that tops the league, getting its dark rich purple colour from anthocyanin, a powerful antioxidant.

* **Cherries** - potent source of anthocyanin, especially sour cherries which also have more Vitamin C than their sweet cherry cousins.

- **Cranberries** - a rich source of antioxidants, they also contain an antibacterial which has been shown to be of help in the treatment of urinary tract infections.

- **Grapes** - a source of manganese and contain resveratrol, an antioxidant thought to help in the prevention of heart disease.

- **Kiwi fruit** - packed with magnesium and potassium as well as the Vitamins C and E, containing more Vitamin C than oranges.

- **Oranges** - contain folate and potassium as well as the Vitamin C they are well known for.

- **Peaches** - high in Vitamin A which can help regulate the immune system and fight infections.

- **Pears** - while not an exceptional source of conventional antioxidants, excel in the phytonutrient category. As a result, pear consumption has now been associated with decreased risk from several common diseases such as heart disease and type 2 diabetes which begin with chronic inflammation and oxidative stress. Pears also contain a combination of soluble and insoluble fibre, found especially in their skins, which not only bind with bile acids as a whole but with a special group called secondary bile acids thereby decreasing their concentration in the intestine and lowering cancer risk.

- **Pineapples** - contain bromelain, a natural enzyme which breaks down protein and aids digestion.

Due to its bromelain content, pineapple juice, used as a marinade, is a good meat tenderiser.

* **Tomatoes** - Tomatoes? Yes. They are actually a fruit variety. They contain lycopene, a powerful antioxidant. Unlike with other fruit and vegetables where nutrients are lessened by the cooking process, the lycopene in tomatoes is actually enhanced by cooking.

7

A few selected recipes

Let me remind you that our journey along the way to regaining normal weight involved a lot of trial and error. The results are given to you here on a plate, so to speak! What are listed here as our preferred recipes for breakfast, lunch and dinner quickly evolved. You may decide to try one or two, or all of them, to find out what suits your own pallet. Just remember that variety is the spice of life!

But, before you read what follows, let me ignite some curiosity in you. Once you achieve the phase where you know what you are doing and know that you are in full control of what you are eating, then you will no longer be afraid of what food does to your weight, and then you will be free to experiment.

Take some well-known ingredients such as onions, garlic, cream, paprika, nutmeg, a variety of cheeses, eggs, smoked chicken, chorizo, salmon, prawns, fennel, broccoli, cauliflower, spinach, tomatoes, avocado, peppers in all their varieties, the list can go on and on. All these basic foods, put together in different combinations can produce some superb meals to delight your palate. You will find there will be no need for bread, potatoes, pasta or rice. You can spend a lifetime wallowing in an orgy of flavours without putting on an ounce of weight. Try it. It is worth it. You are worth it. But if you are interested in tried and tested recipes have a look at these. Each recipe is given to provide for two people unless stated otherwise.

For a selection of these recipes, together with colour photographs of the prepared meals, visit the Panarc Publishing website at www.panarcpublishing.com.

BREAKFAST

Poached eggs on other than toast - quick and easy:

Saucepan of lightly simmering water with a dash of lemon juice or light vinegar

4 eggs

pinch of salt

2 slices of smoked salmon or good quality cold meats, ham or pastrami

Break each egg into a cup and slip gently into the simmering water. Poach for between two to four minutes until the white is fully set. Alternatively a poacher can be used. Lay out your chosen base on two plates. Drain the poached eggs using a slotted spoon and serve on the base.

~

Scrambled eggs with smoked haddock or smoked salmon:

4 eggs

4 tsp single cream

Salt & pepper

good knob of butter

2 fillets of lightly smoked haddock (without colouring) or 2 large slices of smoked salmon

2 tsp chopped chives

Place the haddock in a steamer or poach gently until cooked.

Break the eggs into a bowl, add the cream, salt and pepper to taste. Whisk with a fork until mixed.

Melt some butter in a small saucepan. Add the egg mixture and cook gently, stirring constantly, over a light heat until the eggs are softly set.

Meanwhile, place the fish on two plates. While the eggs are still creamy stir in the chopped chives and pile onto the fish for immediate serving.

Breakfast Omelettes

This is a basic omelette with a variety of fillings.

Basic ingredients:

> *4 eggs*
>
> *4 tsps cream*
>
> *salt & pepper*
>
> *butter or olive oil to cook*
>
> *Fillings:*
>
> *streaky bacon, sliced and fried*
>
> *cooked ham, sliced or cut into cubes*
>
> *smoked haddock, cooked and flaked*
>
> *shrimps, warmed through in a little butter with or without garlic*
>
> *cheddar or other hard cheese grated*
>
> *mushrooms, sliced and fried*
>
> *halved cherry tomatoes, lightly fried*
>
> *herbs – finely chopped*

Break the eggs into a bowl and add the cream, salt and pepper to taste. Stir until well mixed.

Lightly coat an omelette pan or frying pan with a little melted butter or olive oil and pour in the egg mixture. Cook gently until nearly set then add the filling to half the omelette. Fold in half and serve immediately on warmed plates.

The cooking is finished when the omelette sets. It is ready to serve for two.

Baked ham, eggs and tomato

2 beef tomatoes large enough to hold an egg

50 g (2oz) cooked ham

a pinch of chopped herbs

2 eggs

salt & pepper

Cut the tops of the tomatoes and scoop out the seeds and pulp. Separate the seeds from the pulse through a sieve.

Mix the ham, herbs, and season to taste. Divide it in two and fill the tomatoes half way with the mixture.

Place them in a baking dish and break an egg into each of the tomatoes, adding salt and pepper to taste.

Bake in a pre-heated oven at 190°C (gas mark 5) until the eggs set. This should take about 12-15 minutes. Serve hot.

~~~

Kippers and scrambled eggs

2 kipper fillets

4 eggs

single cream

butter to taste

salt and pepper

Wash the kipper fillets well. Place them in a saucepan and cover them with water. Cook gently for about three minutes. Drain on warmed plates with a knob of butter on each.

For a change, the kippers may be fried in olive oil for about 5-6 minutes.

While the kippers are cooking, mix the eggs with a little cream.

Place some butter into a small saucepan and, when melted, add the egg mixture. Stir gently until the eggs have just set but are still moist.

Serve with the kippers and season to taste, being careful with the salt as the kippers are likely to be salty. Serve immediately.

And now for the traditional cooked ENGLISH BREAKFAST.

Select from the following ingredients to suit your appetite:

rashers of bacon

eggs

sausages

slices of black pudding

mushrooms

tomatoes

salt & pepper

The sausages and black pudding contain a quantity of carbohydrates, so avoid adding fried bread, fried potatoes and baked beans.

Fry the bacon, sausages and sliced black pudding. Set aside and keep warm.

Cut the tomatoes in half and fry with the mushrooms until cooked. Remove and keep warm.

Fry the eggs until the whites are firm. Preheat two plates and place half the ingredients on each plate. Season to taste.

~

LUNCH & DINNER

Now let's look at meals for lunch and dinner. There are two scenarios I would like to consider:

- one where lunch consists of a sandwich or a work's canteen meal;
- the other where lunch is prepared in the home.

There is, in fact, one other situation where one has a restaurant meal. I will ignore this scenario because this is a matter of menu selection.

Sandwiches

There was a time, while we were both working, when the standard lunch was made up of sandwiches and fruit. We looked at sandwiches as two separate components; the outside and the fillings. The outside was invariably bread either sliced or in the form of a roll or baguette, that is, carbohydrate. We decided that we would restrict the bread to one slice and satisfy our needs with a variety of fillings. So, we buttered the bread liberally and used one or a combination of the fillings below:

- good slices of roast cold beef with mustard or horse radish, mayonnaise and sliced tomatoes
- minced lamb mixed with a little mint sauce (usually left over from dinner)
- crisply fried bacon and sliced red pepper. Also good with brie or camembert cheese
- grated or sliced hard cheese, such as, cheddar or

Red Leicester with lettuce and mayonnaise
or chutney
* ham and chicken slices, smoked chicken works
particularly well
* toasted cheese and bacon
* scrambled eggs with a little chopped anchovy and
water cress
* smoked salmon peppered and sprinkled with
lemon juice
* sardines with lemon juice, black pepper and
sliced tomato

The list is easily expanded with your favourites, provided the chosen fillings contain very little carbohydrate.

Sometimes, we used up meal left-overs or left-over ingredients to prepare a salad instead of sandwiches. A small plastic (Tupperware) container is ideal both to transport as well as to eat from, just with a fork.

Here are some examples which are easy to prepare and are very filling on a busy day:

* cubes of hard cheese, such as Cheddar, Edam,
Red Leicester, Wensleydale, or whatever is your
favourite, with slices of red pepper, celery, cherry
tomatoes or other salad ingredients
* strips of cooked ham rolled around a soft cheese,
such as, Philadelphia or mascarpone cheese
* chicken legs or hard boiled eggs are also great
favorites with slices of tomatoes, celery or coleslaw

On the following pages I will give you a list of meals which can be eaten for lunch or dinner in any combination, remembering the four basic groups of food ingredients listed earlier. Some of these meals we have enjoyed ourselves. Some of the recipes we have found along the way but have not yet tried. However, because they sound very appetizing and provide the right balance of nutrients, I wanted to include them here. You will be the judge of what interests you and what takes your fancy.

SOUPS

Asparagus and Leek soup

½ litre (1 pint) of chicken stock

340 grams (12 oz) asparagus

1 large leek

2 tablespoon of butter

6 tablespoon of double cream

salt and pepper

These ingredients will make about 4 servings.

Cut off the green end of the leek and cut the stem in half lengths wise. Wash thoroughly and finely chop. Wash the asparagus and chop the tender part of the stalk into small pieces, leaving spears whole.

Melt the butter in a medium size saucepan and add the leeks. Cook for 3-4 minutes stirring often, and then add the asparagus. Cook for a further 1-2 minutes, before adding the chicken stock. Bring to the boil, and then simmer for about 10-11 minutes, or until the asparagus is tender. Add the double cream, season to taste stirring for another minute.

The soup is ready to serve. You can also blend it until smooth and creamy, keeping a few spears whole for a garnish.

Cheese and bacon soup

70 grams (2½ oz) cheddar cheese, grated

5 strips of bacon

8 oz mushrooms sliced

1 leek

½ litre (1 pint) chicken stock

2 tablespoons of butter

salt and pepper

These ingredients would make about 2-3 helpings.

Chop up the bacon into small pieces and fry it until crisp.

Cut off the green part of the leek, cut the white part in two length wise, wash and chop into small pieces.

Grate the cheese.

Heat the butter in a suitable saucepan. When hot, add the leeks and mushrooms and cook them for about five minutes, stirring frequently.

Add the chicken stock and simmer for another 10 minutes.

Transfer the soup into a food processor, add the cheese and process it for about one minute.

Serve immediately, sprinkling the fried bacon bits on top.

Chicken and Egg soup

1 litre (2 pints) chicken stock

200 g (8oz) ground almonds

6 finely chopped chicken breasts or thigh meat

3 round whole meal bread rolls

salt and pepper

6 eggs

These ingredients will make six servings. Adjust for smaller servings.

Bring the stock to the boil. After five minutes add the chicken and the almonds and cook for about 15 minutes.

Meanwhile, halve the bread rolls and scoop out the soft centre. Crisp the shells in the oven.

Strain the soup and stuff the bread rolls with some of the chicken almond mixture. Keep them warm.

Return the remainder of the chicken mix to the soup and puree in a blender. Reheat it and add seasoning to taste.

Poach the eggs.

Serve the soup in bowls and place the rolls and eggs on top of the soup. Serve immediately.

~~~

LUNCHTIME SALADS

Hardly more cumbersome to eat but equally delicious are salads with cold meats such as, boiled bacon, roast beef, sliced roast chicken or drumstick, roast duck, fish, such as tuna, salmon and sardines. Hard boiled eggs, eaten whole or as egg mayonnaise, all may be prepared in easy to eat portions to be consumed with a fork or fingers.

SEAFOOD DISHES

Cod with lemon-parsley sauce

½ kilogram (1.1 lb) cod fillets
120 grams (4 oz) chopped onions
3 cloves of crushed garlic
1 tblspn olive oil
1 tblspn butter
juice of ½ lemon
¾ oz chopped fresh parsley
½ oz chopped fresh thyme
salt and pepper

Heat the butter and olive oil in a frying pan until the butter has melted. Add the onion and fry gently until soft and translucent; then add the garlic and continue frying for about a minute.

Add the cod fillets and fry for about five minutes, turning once.

Add the lemon juice, thyme and parsley and season to taste. Cover the frying pan and cook for a further two minutes.

Serve at once.

These ingredients will serve two.

Trout and pine nuts

285 gr (10 oz) trout fillets

28 gr (1 oz) clarified butter

110 gr (4 oz) unsalted butter

28 gr (1 oz) lightly toasted pine nuts

1 tbsp chopped fresh parsley

1 tbsp chopped chives

2 tbsp lemon juice

plain flour for dredging

salt and pepper

Season the trout fillets with salt and pepper and dredge them in flour. Shake the excess flour off.

Add the clarified butter to a large frying pan till the butter is hot but not smoking. Add the trout fillets, skin side up fry them for about two minutes. Turn the fillets and fry for a further two minutes. Place on warmed plates.

Add the butter and the pine nuts and continue frying, swirling the content until the butter begins to brown.

Remove from heat and stir in the lemon juice, the chives and parsley, add salt to taste.

Spoon the liquid over the trout fillets and serve.

These ingredients should serve 3 - 4.

Stuffed courgettes with prawns

4 medium sized courgettes

14 gr (½ oz) butter

226 gr (8 oz) prawns

2 tbsp lemon juice

lemon slices, for serving

black pepper

Boil the courgettes in salt water for about 10 minutes. Take them out of the water and put aside.

Place the butter in a frying pan. When melted, add the prawns and gently heat through.

Slice the courgettes lengthwise and fill them with the prawns. Sprinkle with lemon juice and black pepper and garnish with lemon slices.

These ingredients should serve two.

Prawns au gratin

226 gr (8 oz) prawns

85 gr (3 oz) grated cheddar or red Leicester cheese

2 large red onions, finely chopped

250 ml (8 fluid oz) double cream

1oz butter plus extra for greasing

salt and black pepper

Grease four individual gratin dishes.

Fry the onions in the butter until soft and translucent. Remove the onions with a slotted spoon and place in the four gratin dishes.

Wash the prawns thoroughly, dry with kitchen paper and stir into the remaining butter, adding them to the dishes.

Season to taste with black pepper.

Pre-heat a grill to medium-high setting. Pour the cream over the gratin dishes then sprinkle them with the cheese. Grill for about 5 minutes or until the cheese starts bubbling.

These ingredients should serve four.

POULTRY DISHES

Paprika chicken

(Hungarian favourite of mine)

6 chicken thighs

2 medium sized onions chopped

1 medium red pepper chopped

3 medium tomatoes chopped

2 cloves of crushed garlic

3 oz goose fat or olive oil

100 ml white wine

100 ml chicken stock or water

150 ml sour cream

1½ tbsp. sweet paprika

1 pinch of hot paprika (optional)

salt

Heat the goose fat or olive oil in a saucepan large enough to take all the ingredients. Add the chopped onions and peppers and fry gently until tender. Add the garlic and cook for a further minute stirring occasionally.

Take off the heat and add the paprika and tomatoes. Stir the mixture well before adding the chicken pieces, coating them well with the mixture.

Add the chicken stock and the wine and put back on the heat. If needed, add a little water to make sure that the chicken pieces are almost covered. Cover the saucepan and simmer for about 30 minutes, or until the meat is tender. Uncover the saucepan and cook for another 10 minutes to reduce the sauce. Check the seasoning and serve topped with a spoonful or two of soured cream per portion.

These ingredients should serve 3 people.

Chicken and Mushrooms.

4 boneless chicken thighs or 2 small
chicken breasts

8oz. mushrooms sliced

1 oz. minced shallots

1½ oz. butter

100 ml chicken stock

100 ml white wine

150 ml double cream

1 oz. fresh parsley

1 teaspoon fresh thyme

salt and pepper

Cut the chicken meat to about 20mm (3/4") slices. Season the slices with thyme, salt and pepper.

Heat the butter in a frying pan and fry the chicken pieces until golden.

Add the mushrooms and fry for about another 2-3 minutes. Remove the chicken-mushroom mixture and put aside.

Add the shallots to the pan and fry for 2-3 minutes, stirring occasionally.

Add the chicken stock and wine and simmer for about five minutes on a medium heat. Stir to dissolve the sediment from the bottom of the frying pan before adding the cream and simmer for another five minutes.

Finally replace the chicken and mushroom mix together with the parsley into the pan and simmer for a further 2-3 minutes until the chicken is heated through.

Season to taste and serve immediately with a vegetable, such as broccoli or cauliflower.

These ingredients should serve two.

Duck breast with cognac or orange juice.

1 large whole duck breast

1 knob of butter or duck fat

1 small wineglass of cognac

juice of one orange

salt and pepper

Pre-heat the oven to 215 degrees C. Wash the duck breast and dry with kitchen paper. Score the skin side diagonally, making a diamond pattern, taking care not to cut into the meat. Very lightly grease a medium sized frying pan and heat.

Place the duck breast into the frying pan skin side down and fry on a medium heat until most of the fat has run out of the breast and the skin becomes golden brown. Turn the duck meat side down briefly in the hot fat and then remove it from the frying pan, placing it skin side up into an oven proof dish.

Drain the duck fat from the frying pan and reserve for cooking. Add the cognac and orange juice and deglaze the pan. Pour the mixture round the duck breast and well season the duck skin.

Place into the preheated oven and cook for 10 -12 minutes. This will leave the meat pink.

Remove from the oven and leave to rest for 5-6 minutes before slicing and serving. Add any meat juice to the sauce and divide between the plates.

One large duck breast should serve 2 people.

MEAT DISHES

Ham with cream of port sauce.

2 thick slices of cooked ham, about 6 oz. each

1tbspn butter

3 tbspn minced shallots

4 fluid oz white wine

3 tbspn port wine

1 tspn tomato paste

4 fluid oz double cream

salt and pepper

Heat the butter in a frying pan until hot. Add the shallots and fry for about two minutes or until translucent. Add the wine and port wine to the frying pan and bring to the boil before adding the ham. Simmer for about 3-4 minutes. Remove the ham from the frying pan and keep warm.

Whisk the tomato paste and cream together and add to the frying pan. Bring to the boil and simmer for about four minutes, stirring frequently. Season with salt and pepper.

Place the ham slices onto two serving plates and pour the sauce over them.

Serve immediately.

These ingredients serve two people.

Caribbean beef pot roast.

4 pieces of braising steak about 250gms (½ lb) each

30gms beef dripping or clarified butter

3 tbsp rum

8 chopped pimento-stuffed olives

2 tbsp tomato paste

salt and pepper

Heat the lard or butter in a frying pan until hot. Brown the steaks on all sides. Pour off the fat and add the rum to the frying pan. Cover the frying pan tightly and simmer the meat for 20 minutes.

Stir in the tomato paste, add salt and pepper to taste and continue to simmer for another two hours. Check occasionally and add some boiling water to the pan if there is a danger of it running dry.

When the cooking time is up, check that the meat is tender before serving it on four plates. Skim the fat off the liquid in the frying pan and stir in the olives.

Reheat and spoon the sauce over the meat.

These ingredients will serve four people.

Beef goulash.

450gr.(1 lb.) cubed stewing steak

60gr (2 oz) fat bacon

half stick of chorizo

30gr. (1oz.) lard or clarified butter

150ml (5 fluid oz.) beef stock

2 finely chopped large onions

2 crushed garlic cloves

1 glass red wine

1 bouquet garni

salt and 1 tblspn of sweet paprika pepper

In a medium sized saucepan heat the lard or butter until hot. Chop the bacon and chorizo coarsely and add to the pan together with the onion and fry stirring frequently, for about five minutes. Add the garlic and stir.

Remove from the heat and stir in the paprika. Add the meat cubes to the saucepan. Stir well until all the meat is covered. Add the wine, the stock and the *bouquet garni*. Season liberally with salt, pepper and simmer for 1½-2 hours.

Remove the bouquet of garni and serve on three plates.

These ingredients serve three.

Pork medallions with sour cream and dill.

½kg (1 lb.) pork tenderloin sliced into six slices

2 tbsp butter

120 ml (4 fluid oz.) chicken stock

1 clove of crushed garlic

1 tbsp cognac

60ml (2 fluid oz.) soured cream

½ tsp white pepper

1 tsp chopped fresh dill

salt

Heat the butter in a heavy frying pan until hot. Add the pork medallion slices and fry them on both sides for five minutes or until nice and brown. Remove the pork slices and keep warm.

Add the chicken stock, cognac and garlic and stir the mixture, making sure that the caramelised fat at the bottom of the pan is well incorporated. Reduce for about 2-3 minutes. Remove the frying pan from the heat and add the soured cream spoonful by spoonful carefully stirring each into the mixture.

Return the pork to the frying pan, including any juices left on the plate. Cook the meat for 2-3 more minutes on medium heat. Place the pork slices onto two serving plates and pour the sauce over them. Sprinkle with pepper and dill.

These ingredients serve two people.

Piperade or Lecsó

This is a delicious stew of onions, peppers, tomatoes, garlic and egg, flavoured with spicy chorizo. For vegetarians, simply omit the chorizo and replace with hot paprika to taste.

2 medium sized onions

4 red or yellow peppers

5 medium sized tomatoes

3 cloves of garlic

4 eggs

Olive oil

Salt

1 ring chorizo (hot)

Method:

Chop the onions, peppers and tomatoes into bite size pieces. Crush the garlic and slice the chorizo. Heat a little olive oil in a frying pan or saucepan large enough to take all the ingredients.

Place the chopped peppers and onions into the pan together with the chorizo and fry gently until the vegetables are tender and the chorizo has released all its flavoured oils. (If you are preparing the non-vegetarian version, omit the chorizo and add paprika at this stage.)

Stir in the garlic and add the tomatoes. Stir again gently to make sure all the ingredients are combined, cover and simmer for about 30 minutes. Season to taste with salt and extra paprika if desired.

Remove from the heat and add the beaten eggs, stirring all the time as they cook and thicken the stew. Alternatively, poach them separately and place one on top of each serving.

These ingredients serve four.

8

Get on with it

So, finally, it is over to you. You now know about the nutrients in food and the best time to consume those nutrients. Now you can create your own eating plan to suit you and decide what you are going to enjoy for breakfast, lunch and dinner each day in order to shed that excess weight. In a word, you can escape from obesity, take control of your weight and retain your normal weight for the rest of your life.

In Appendix 1, I list some of the common food ingredients found in our shopping trollies, giving the carbohydrate content in an average serving.

When creating a plan of action for yourself it should contain some or all of the following measures.

- Do not buy any foods that provide mainly energy with little or no nutrients. This means sugar first of all and sugar in biscuits, cakes and other attractive looking confectionary. That way money can be saved to spend on better quality foods.

- Do not buy manufactured foods or drinks that are marked as 'low fat', 'fat free' or 'low cholesterol' products. That includes manufactured sauces that contain high levels of high fructose corn syrup, skimmed milk and low fat dairy products.

- Do not buy or use margarines.

- Do not use vegetable based oils if they are to be heated before being consumed. Olive oil is an exception to this rule.

- Do not buy processed, ready-made and manufactured foods and drinks which contain high levels of sugar and salt.

- Do not buy fizzy drinks regardless whether they contain sugar or artificial sweeteners and beware of pure fruit juices. Check their sugar content. Even fruit juices with no added sugar contain many spoonsful of sugar in the form of high fructose corn syrup.

- Buy fresh fruit not fruit juice. Make your own fruit juice.

- Buy only fresh vegetables.

- Use saturated fats, such as butter, lard, duck fat and goose fat for cooking and in food. Olive oil may also be used.

- Buy fresh meat or poultry and prepare them yourself.

- Whenever possible prepare the meals you eat yourself so that you know exactly what you are putting in your mouth and can enjoy without fear.

- Avoid eating between meals. If you must, have a small piece of hard cheese, a handful of almonds or Brazil nuts or full fat natural yoghurt.
- Do not have biscuits or cakes with your coffee or tea.
- Enjoy a variety of new flavours once you have done away with your current addiction to sweet foods and re-educated your taste buds.
- Always be ready to experiment with new flavours to enhance the enjoyment of eating.
- Remember, an occasional digression from your normal way of eating, such as in a restaurant or when having dinner with friends will not interfere with your weight loss provided it is an occasional digression only.
- Be aware of the portions of food you put on your plate. Reduce the portions you serve yourself as you proceed with your plan of reducing weight.
- Finally, always be guided by your appetite and stop eating when it signals that you have eaten enough.

All there is left to be said is: "Go for it". Take control and enjoy every minute of the rest of your life with your normal weight, greater vitality and pain free days to come.

Good luck.

Appendix 1

Alphabetical list of some foods and their carbohydrate content in popular average portions

Meat, fish, eggs, cheese, butter, margarine, fats and oils contain no carbohydrate and are therefore not included in this list.

Food and drink items	Portion in once	metric	Carbs in grams
Ale, light	½ pint	284 ml	25
strong	½ pint	284 ml	30
All bran	½ oz	14 gr	7.5
Almonds	30 nuts		2.5
Apple fruit	1.4 oz	40 gr	10
Apple juice	8 oz	227 gr	20
Apple pie	4 oz	115 gr	35
Apricot fruit	1.2 oz	34 gr	5
In syrup	4 oz	115 gr	25
Apricot dry	1 oz	28 gr	10
Artichokes	5 oz	142 gr	5
Asparagus	4 oz	115 gr	2.5
Avocado pear	½ oz	14 gr	5

Food and drink items	Portion in once	metric	Carbs in grams
Banana	1.4 oz	40gr	25
Barley, cooked	3 oz	85 gr	20
Beans, baked	4 oz	115 gr	20
broad	4 oz	115 gr	15
green	4 oz	115 gr	2.5
Haricot cooked	4 oz	115 gr	20
Beer, light	½ pint	284 ml	25
heavy	½ pint	284 ml	35
Beetroot	2 oz	57 gr	5
Biscuit, sweet	2 small		15
plain	3 medium		15
Bitter lemon	6 oz	170 ml	20
Blackberries raw	4 oz	115 gr	10
Blackcurrants	2 oz	57 gr	5
Blackcurrant syrup	1 oz	28 gr	17½
Black pudding	2 oz	57 gr	15
Bournvita	½ oz	14 gr	14
Bovril	½ oz	14 gr	0
Brandy	1 oz	28 gr	20
Brazil nuts	10 nuts		2.5
Bread 1 slice	1 oz	28 gr	15
Bread starch reduced	1 oz	28 gr	10
Buckwheat cooked	3 oz	85 gr	20
Bun, plain	2 oz	57 gr	25
Bun, fruit	2 oz	57 gr	30
Bun, ice sugared	2 oz	57 gr	40
Butter beans	2 oz	57 gr	15
Cabbage	4 oz	115 gr	½
Cakes, plain	2 oz	57 gr	35
Cakes, cream	2 oz	57 gr	35
Cakes, rich fruit	2 oz	57 gr	40
Carrot	3 oz	85 gr	5
Cashew nuts	1 oz	28 gr	10

Food and drink items	Portion in once	metric	Carbs in grams
Cauliflower	4 oz	115 gr	½
Celery	4 oz	115 gr	½
Cherries	4 oz	115 gr	15
Chestnuts	2 oz	57 gr	20
Chocolate	2 oz	57 gr	25
Chocolate drink	8 oz	227 gr	30
Chutney	½ oz	14 gr	5
Cider	½ pint	284 ml	35
Coca Cola	6 oz	170 ml	15
Cocoa powder	1 teaspoon		0
Coconut, fresh	1 oz	28gr	7.5
Coffee, black	1 cup		0
Corn, canned	4 oz	115 gr	20
Corn on the cob	1 cob		20
Cornflakes	¾ oz	21 gr	20
Cornflour	1 oz	28 gr	25
Cottage cheese	2 oz	57 gr	½
Cottage pie	4 oz	115 gr	15
Cranberries	2 oz	57 gr	5
Cranberry sauce	1 oz	28 gr	12.5
Cream	1 oz	28 gr	0
Cucumber	2 oz	57 gr	0
Currants, black, red	2 oz	57 gr	5
Custard	4 oz	115 gr	10
Damsons	2 oz	57 gr	5
Dates	1 oz	28 gr	20
Doughnuts	2 oz	57 gr	30
Energen crisp bread	1 piece		½
Figs, fresh	2 oz	57 gr	7.5
Figs, dried	1 oz	28 gr	15
Figs in syrup	4 oz	115 gr	40
Fish cake	2 oz	57 gr	10

Food and drink items	Portion in once	metric	Carbs in grams
Flour, barley	1 oz	28 gr	20
Flour, corn	1 oz	28 gr	25
Flour, oat	1 oz	28 gr	20
Flour, wheat	1 oz	28 gr	20
Gin	1 oz	28 gr	20
Ginger beer	8 oz	227 gr	30
Glucose	1 oz	28 gr	30
Gooseberries	4 oz	115 gr	10
Gooseberries in syrup	4 oz	115 gr	25
Grapefruit	4 oz	115 gr	5
Grapefruit juice	4 oz	115 gr	15
Grapes	4 oz	115 gr	15
Greengages	4 oz	115 gr	12.5
Haggis	4 oz	115 gr	20
Hazel nuts	15 nuts		2.5
Honey	1 oz	28 gr	25
Horlicks	1 tablespoon		10
Ice cream	1 oz	28 gr	15
Irish stew	4 oz	115 gr	10
Jam	½ oz	14 gr	10
Jelly	4 oz	115 gr	20
Junket	4 oz	115 gr	15
Kedgeree	4 oz	115 gr	25
Kiwi fruit	1 fruit		6
Kohlrabi	4 oz	115 gr	5
Lager	½ pint	284 ml	20
Lancashire hot pot	6 oz	170 gr	15

Food and drink items	Portion in once	metric	Carbs in grams
Leeks	4 oz	115 gr	5
Lemonade	8oz	227 ml	25
Lentils, cooked	4 oz	115 gr	30
Liqueurs, sweet	1 oz	28 ml	25
Loganberries	4 oz	115 gr	5
Loganberries in syrup	4 oz	115 gr	30
Lucozade	6 oz	170 ml	30
Macaroni, cooked	6 oz	170 gr	50
Macaroni cheese	4 oz	115 gr	25
Macvita	1 piece		12.5
Mandarin	4 oz	115 gr	10
Mango	6 oz	170 gr	20
Marmalade	½ oz	14 gr	10
Marmite	½ oz	14 gr	0
Marrow	4 oz	115 gr	0
Mayonnaise	½ oz	14 gr	0
Melon	6 oz	170 gr	10
Milk	½ pint	284 ml	15
Milk pudding	4 oz	115 gr	25
Mince pie	2 oz	57 gr	25
Molasses	1 oz	28 gr	20
Mulberries	4 oz	115 gr	10
Mushrooms	2 oz	57 gr	0
Nectarines	4 oz	115 gr	15
Noodles cooked	6 oz	170 gr	45
Nuts, shelled	1 oz	28 gr	2.5
Oat cakes	1 oz	28 gr	15
Oatmeal, uncooked	1 oz	28 gr	15
Olives	1 oz	28 gr	0
Onion	1 oz	28gr	0
Orange	6 oz	170 gr	15

Food and drink items	Portion in once	metric	Carbs in grams
Orange juice sweet	4 oz	113 ml	10
Ovaltine	1 tablespoon		5
Pancakes	2 oz	57 gr	20
Parsnip	4 oz	115 gr	10
Passion fruit, raw	2 oz	57 gr	5
Pastry, cooked	1 oz	28 gr	15
Pawpaw	6 oz	170 gr	10
Peach, raw	1.5 oz	42 gr	10
Peach in syrup	4oz	115 gr	20
Peanut	30 nuts		5
Peanut butter	1 oz	28 gr	5
Pear, fruit	1.5 oz	42 gr	12.5
Pear in syrup	4 oz	115 gr	20
Peas, green	4 oz	115 gr	10
Peas, dried	1 oz	28 gr	20
Pineapple fruit	4 oz	115 gr	10
Pineapple in syrup	4 oz	115 gr	25
Plums, fruit	4 oz	115 gr	10
Plums, in syrup	4 oz	115 gr	20
Plum pudding	3 oz	85 gr	45
Port wine	2 oz	56 ml	23
Potatoes	3 oz	85 gr	15
Potato crisps	1 oz	28 gr	15
Prunes, dried	1 oz	28 gr	5
Raisins	1 oz	28 gr	20
Raspberries, fruit	4 oz	115 gr	10
Raspberries in syrup	4 oz	115 gr	30
Redcurrants	4 oz	115 gr	5
Rhubarb	4 oz	115 gr	0
Rhubarb pie	4 oz	115 gr	30
Ribena	1 oz	28 ml	17.5
Rice cooked	4 oz	115 gr	20

Food and drink items	Portion in once	metric	Carbs in grams
Rice pudding	4 oz	115 gr	25
Roll, bread	2 oz	87 gr	30
Rita	1 piece		7.5
Sago pudding	4 oz	115 gr	20
Salad dressing	½ oz	14 ml	½
Sausage, with cereals	3 oz	85 gr	10
Sausage, all meat	3 oz	85 gr	0
Scone	2 oz	87 gr	30
Scotch broth	8 oz	227 ml	7.5
Semolina uncooked	1 oz	28gr	20
Semolina pudding	4 oz	115 gr	20
Sherry	2 oz	85 ml	20
Soups	8 oz	227 ml	10
Spaghetti cooked	6 oz	170 gr	50
Spaghetti in tomato sauce	4 oz	115 gr	15
Steak and kidney pie	4 oz	115 gr	20
Stout	½ pint	284 ml	35
Strawberries	4 oz	115 gr	7.5
Sugar	½ oz	14 gr	15
Sultanas	1 oz	28 gr	20
Swedes	4 oz	115 gr	5
Sweets	1 oz	28 gr	20
Sweet potatoes	3 oz	85 gr	25
Syrup, golden	½ oz	14 ml	7.5
Tangerines	3 oz	85 gr	10
Tapioca, cooked	4 oz	115 gr	20
Tapioca pudding	4 oz	115 gr	25
Tea, without milk	1 cup		0
Tinned fruit in syrup	4 oz	115 gr	25
Tinned fruit juice	5 oz	142 ml	25
Tomato	4 oz	115 gr	5
Tomato juice	5 oz	142 ml	5

Food and drink items	Portion in once	metric	Carbs in grams
Tonic water	6 oz	170 ml	15
Treacle	½ oz	14 gr	7.5
Turnip	3 oz	85 gr	5
Vermicelli, cooked	2 oz	85 gr	45
Vermouth, dry	2 oz	85 ml	15
Vermouth, sweet	2 oz	85 ml	25
Vinegar			0
Vinegar, balsamic			1
Vita-wheat	1 piece		7.5
Walnuts	10 nuts		2.5
Wheat germ	½ oz	14gr	7.5
Whisky	1 oz	28 gr	20
Wines, dry	3 oz	85 ml	15
Wines sweet	3 oz	85 ml	20
Yam	4 oz	115 gr	20
Yeast dried	½ oz	14 gr	5
Yoghurt plain	5 oz	142 ml	10
Yoghurt flavoured	6 oz	170 ml	20
Yorkshire pudding	2 oz	85 gr	15

Appendix 2

A simple A to Z of useful definitions

'A'

Absorption is a process by which the nutrients in consumed and digested food, passes through the wall of the gut into the blood stream.

Addiction is normally understood to relate to the use of drugs, nicotine and alcoholic drinks. In relation to obesity, addiction can develop to certain flavours, such as, sweetness or to textures of food. This addiction can be characterised as a physical or psychological dependence which demonstrates as an uncontrollable desire or craving. As an increased tolerance is built up, more and more of the chosen food is required to produce the same level of satisfaction.

Alcohol is made by the fermentation of glucose by yeast. In the body the oxidation of alcohol produces energy similar to that of sugar. Alcoholic beverages come in many familiar forms from beer to vodka, cider to champagne. Alcohol is a stimulant in small doses and a depressant in large ones. Over consumption comes with a range of health problems, such as, liver damage, cancer and heart disease.

Amino-acids are constituent compounds of proteins. Our body requires protein as a nutrient because the amino-acids metabolised from it are the building blocks of our cells. Also, amino-acids play an important role in the building of the central nervous system as well as keeping the body's immune system functioning. The best food sources of the essential amino-acids are first class proteins such as meat and fish. Pulses and grains contain a variety of second class proteins.

Antioxidants, as the name suggests, are substances that prevent or retard oxidation. Oxygen is essential to life, but as our bodies use oxygen, we generate by-products known as free radicals. Although a normal part of the body's response, they can damage healthy cells. Antioxidants neutralise the effect of free radicals. The body produces a range of its own protective antioxidants, but some foods are also rich in them and these may boost the body's own supply. Two of the best known are Vitamin C which is soluble in water and vitamin E which is fat soluble. Their effects can be demonstrated outside of the body as Vitamin C (in the form of lemon juice) prevents the browning of cut fruit, (apples for example), whilst Vitamin E is used to reduce the rancidity of fats.

'B'

Baking is a process of cooking using dry heat. Most often associated with the making of bread.

Balanced diet is one which provides the right amount of food for your daily activities and to maintain your body processes through a whole variety of food sources providing protein, fat, carbohydrate, vitamins and trace elements.

Beta-carotene is a yellow/orange pigment which gives vegetables that colour. Indeed the name carotene comes from the word 'carrot'. Beta-carotene is converted by the human body into Vitamin A, which we need for good eye health, our immune systems as well as a healthy skin and mucous membranes. Beta-carotene itself is not an essential nutrient but Vitamin A is.

Bile is a greenish liquid produced in the liver and stored in the gall bladder. It aids the digestion of fats in the small intestine.

Body fat is stored in living cells called adipose tissues and serves a number of vital functions. Created from glucose by insulin, it stores energy for use when food is not available, conserves body heat and provides body contour. When body fat breaks down into fatty acids to be oxidised in the blood stream this process is controlled by hormones including insulin and adrenaline.

'C'

Calcium is an important mineral element in the body. Most of it resides in the bones, but some must be present in the blood stream and soft tissues. Here, calcium plays a role in blood clotting, functioning of the nervous system and muscles. Good food sources of calcium are dairy products such as milk and cheese.

Calorie is a unit of heat energy. It is associated with measuring the energy content of the various foods we eat. Maintaining a preferred weight using calorie counting is often abridged to 'calories in should equal calories out'.

Carbohydrates are technically hydrates of carbon and are formed in plants, by synthesising glucose from water and carbon dioxide. In food science carbohydrate refers to any food which is rich in complex carbohydrates, such as bread, cereals and pasta or simple carbohydrates such as sugar which is found in desserts, jams and sweets.

Carotene (see Beta-carotene)

Cereals - There are about seven major cereals available for food production. They are wheat, rice, corn, millet, barley, rye and oats. A vast range of foods and drinks are made from these. They represent the main sources of starches in our food.

Cheese is made of milk mainly from cows, sheep and goats. Milk is separated into curds and whey by the use of an enzyme such as rennet. It is the curds which are used to form the vast variety of cheeses available today. Protein, fat, vitamins and calcium from the milk are concentrated in the cheese to form a highly nutritious food. This is especially the case in hard cheeses.

Cholesterol is a white waxy material mainly found in animal tissue. It is vital for the body as it produces a range of substances, such as bile salts, cortisol, vitamin D and the sex hormones. Also, cholesterol is a 'building or repair' substance as it creates or repairs the membranes of cells. The amount of cholesterol at any given time is very accurately controlled in a healthy body. It is mainly synthesised in the liver only a small percentage coming from food sources so dietary cholesterol only slightly alters the level in the body as the liver compensates for the intake from food.

Citrus fruit - The fruits which belong to this category are noted for their high juice content and characteristic sharp flavour produced by the citric acid they contain. The sharpest are lemon, lime and kumquat while the wide range of oranges and mandarins contain more sugar and are, therefore, more palatable so are widely eaten as raw fruit. All citrus fruits are used in cooking and drunk as juices. Nutritionally they are prized for their levels of vitamin C.

Cobalt is a constituent element of vitamin B12 and is an important dietary trace element. It is toxic in large amounts which is why it is not available in supplement form in the UK. Only tiny amounts are required daily and can be obtained from foods such as fish, oysters, clams, leafy green vegetables, milk, nuts and meat.

Cocoa and chocolate are consumed as chocolate confectionary with the addition of sugar and cocoa butter. Cocoa powder is used in cooking and chocolate drinks.

Cod liver oil is extracted from the livers of Atlantic cod, as the name suggests. It is an essential oil rich in omega 3 fatty acids as well as vitamins A and D. In many countries it is used as a remedy against rickets. As well it is thought to aid joint stiffness and have a beneficial effect on the cardiovascular system. Benefits also extend to the teeth, skin, hair and nails.

Cooking fats - Artificially manufactured cooking fats are made from plant based oils through a process of hydrogenation. If preferred they can be used as a substitute for saturated animal fats such as lard and butter, but when heated they break down to their constituent elements among them trans fats. Not recommended.

Cooking oils - There are a variety of plant based oils which have culinary uses. Among the polyunsaturated oils are sunflower and soybean. All polyunsaturated oils are best used cold as they become chemically unstable when heated. Monounsaturated oils are more stable and can be used in a variety of ways. The best known is olive oil widely lauded as part of the healthy 'Mediterranean' diet.

Copper is an essential trace mineral element found in all body tissues and, together with iron, plays an essential part in the formation of red blood cells. It effects the functioning of the heart, and promotes healthy bones and connective tissue. Good food sources are shell fish, vegetables, especially mushrooms and avocados, nuts, seeds and whole grains.

Cream is produced by the separation of fat from the milk by a process of centrifugation. This involves the spinning of the milk at high speed by an electric motor until the fat globules separate from the heavier liquid. The cream is then pasteurised to kill off any bacteria. The definitions of single, whipping, double and so on refer to the fat content in the finished product.

'D'

Dates are a very sweet fruit, originating from hot countries in the Middle East and North Africa. They are usually consumed in dried form, but in some countries are ground into flour and used in cooking.

Diabetes is a condition where the amount of glucose in the blood is too high because the body cannot utilise it properly as fuel. This occurs when the pancreas produces no insulin (Type 1 diabetes). When there is insufficient insulin or it is not working properly it is Type 2 diabetes. If the insulin is being produced but not working properly it is known as insulin resistance.

Diet is the name for your normal pattern of consumption of food and drink. This is often confused with 'dieting' which is, of course, the consumption of food and drink in a specific regime to achieve a particular outcome, such as weight control.

Dietary requirements - The amount of energy and nutrients required to assure the optimal health and functioning of a person constitute their dietary requirements. The energy requirements are those that maintain an individual's metabolic processes and their day to day physical activities. The requirements for nutrients are given in the form of recommended daily intakes of fat, protein, carbohydrate, vitamins and mineral trace elements.

Digestive juices - The digestive system is composed of secretions that are largely responsible for breaking down food. These are known as the digestive juices. Saliva, which starts the process in the mouth while chewing, turns starches into sugar. The food is then swallowed and enters the stomach and the gastric juices there – primarily hydrochloric acid – continue the process with pepsin and rennin which beak protein down into tiny units. The food continues its journey through the duodenum where two digestive juices are released; pancreatic juice and bile or gall juice which is known to emulsify fats so that they can be absorbed by the intestines. Both the pancreatic and bile juices are alkaline in nature which balances out the whole of the digestive system. In the intestines the food is further subjected to another digestive fluid, succus entericus, which breaks down macromolecules of fat and protein and aids the absorption of vital nutrients.

Dyspepsia is commonly known as indigestion, causing pain, nausea and heartburn, after the consumption of food. Few people have never suffered from indigestion at sometime, but if persistent it could be the sign of something more serious.

'E'

Eggs are a most beneficial food for human consumption. Besides fat, protein and iron, they contain vitamins A, D, E and B.

Energy - The human body requires energy to enable the metabolic processes to take place, to fuel growth, to repair cells and to provide energy for all physical and mental activities. Energy is derived from the precisely controlled oxidation of food. It is, therefore, important to know how much energy is contained in the food that is consumed. As food is oxidised in the body, the energy that is released produces heat. How much energy is provided by a specific food ingredient can be calculated by measuring the heat that it produces. This is done in a calorimeter.

Enzymes act as catalysts in the body promoting the many thousands of processes that take place there. Enzymes are proteins created by living cells. A good example is a digestive enzyme, salivary amylase, which helps to turn starches, such as bread, into a sugar, called, maltose, while the starch is being chewed and mixed with saliva.

Essential nutrients are substances that provide structural or functional components or energy to the body. However, the body cannot make them in sufficient quantity itself so they have to come from the diet. In terms of food ingredients, we refer to essential fatty acids and essential amino acids as well as essential vitamins and trace elements.

'F'

Fat in food is either primarily saturated animal fats, such as dripping, lard and butter; plant based oils such as soybean or conola oil which are primarily polyunsaturated or monounsaturated oils such as olive oil. Not all saturated fats are animal fats. Coconut oil and palm oil are also high in saturates. Fats are basically triglycerides, that is, compounds of glycerol and fatty acids. Dietary fats also contain fat-soluble vitamins A, D, E and K.

Fermentation is a process where micro-organisms act on carbohydrates with little or no oxygen present. The two best known fermentation processes are alcoholic and lactic. Lactic fermentation turns milk into yoghurt. Alcoholic turns fruit into wine with the help of yeast. Another well-known fermented food is cabbage which we eat as sauerkraut.

Fibre - Dietary fibre, or roughage, refers to a group of substances in plant food which cannot be completely broken down by digestive enzymes. Soluble fibre is found in such foods as fruits and beans and it helps you to feel satiated. Insoluble fibre is found in bran, nuts and vegetables and it aids the passage of food, keeping the digestive system regular. In particular, it controls the rate of intestinal carbohydrate absorption.

Fizzy or soft drinks - There are two basic types of manufactured drinks, those which are made with water and those which are based on fruit juices. Invariably they are sweet as they contain many teaspoons of sugar or artificial sweeteners. Those which are prepared by forcing carbon dioxide into the flavoured and sweetened liquid are known as 'fizzy drinks'. Almost all of them provide only empty calories.

Folic acid is part of the water soluble B vitamin complex. The human body needs folate (synthesised from folic acid) to synthesise and repair DNA and it is important in aiding rapid cell growth as in pregnancy and infancy. Both children and adults need folate to produce healthy red blood cells and protect against anaemia. A notable effect of deficiency in pregnancy is neural tube abnormalities in developing embryos. Folic acid is found in many foods, especially in green vegetables and liver.

Food Additives – These substances are added to food for several reasons by manufacturers as well as cooks in their own kitchens. The objectives are enhancing flavour, texture, colour and preservation. In the domestic kitchen additives such as salt, herbs and spices are used to add flavour to the food. Commercially additives are used not only to add flavour but to enhance appearance and give a longer shelf life. For example, there are anti-caking agents, anti-foaming agents, bulking agents and humectants which prevent food from drying out. All legal additives are given a number which in Europe is preceded by the letter 'E'.

Food preservation - there is a variety of ways to preserve food. Some of these have developed over many centuries. Preservatives can be chemical or physical. For example, using acetic acid to reduce the pH level to the point where micro-organisms cannot grow. This method of preservation has been used to produce pickled cucumbers, cabbage and other vegetables for centuries. Meat and fish have been preserved by salting and drying for generations. Canning and freezing are more modern methods of food preservation.

Fructose is a sugar found naturally in fruits, vegetables and honey. It is sweeter than sugar and is metabolised very differently. The burden of its metabolism falls on the liver in a similar way to alcohol. Excessive consumption, as in for example high fructose corn syrup, can create new fat cells in the heart, liver and digestive organs.

'G'

Gall-bladder is a pear shaped hollow structure housed under the liver. It holds and concentrates the bile that the liver produces. When the small intestine is stimulated by food reaching it the gall-bladder squeezes bile through the bile duct into the small intestine to emulsify fats and neutralise acids in the partially digested food.

Gelatine is a mixture of peptides and proteins, derived from collagen. Skin, bones and connective tissue of animals are the best sources of gelatine, for example, pig's head or trotters. Gelatine is dissolved in hot water and will set as a jelly at room temperature. It is used in the preparation of many foods from aspic to marshmallows.

Glucose is a carbohydrate and a monosaccharide or simple sugar. The oxidation or metabolism of glucose contributes to a series of complex biochemical reactions which provide the energy used by cells.

Gluten is a protein found in the cereals wheat, rye and barley. A similar protein is found in oats. The presence of gluten in flour gives bread in all its forms its familiar texture. When the flour is mixed with water and yeast then kneaded the dough becomes elastic trapping the bubbles of carbon dioxide produced by the yeast fermentation in the process.

Glycogen - The brain and other tissues require a constant supply of glucose. Glycogen is a polysaccharide and it is the main storage form of glucose in humans and animals. The highest concentration is found in the liver whilst a far lower concentration is housed in muscle tissue although the overall total in the muscles exceeds that in the liver. This is used during strenuous activity. Smaller amounts are found in the kidneys and white blood cells.

'H'

Herbs and spices - Both, herbs and spices are used as food additives that enhance the flavour of a meal. There are essential oils in these products that impart flavour to the food. Herbs are normally the leaves of edible aromatic plants. Spices are derived from bark, fruit, nuts and flowers.

Honey is made by bees from the nectar of flowers. Nectar is mainly sucrose and water. Bees add enzymes which convert the sucrose into fructose and glucose and evaporate the water. Because of the high level of fructose, honey is sweeter than sugar. Unlike sugar, honey contains small quantities of B group vitamins and amino acids as well as the minerals copper, calcium, iron, magnesium and potassium among others. One of the oldest and completely natural food ingredients still used to day, it contains antioxidants and has antibacterial properties. Honey has been given a whole range of health benefits in folklore.

Hormones are the body's chemical messengers, produced by endocrine glands they travel via the bloodstream to where they are needed in the body. They are used to affect growth, metabolism, sexual function and mood.

'I'

Inflammation occurs when the body suffers some form of irritation or damage. This can be either external or internal. Inflammation is the body's attempt to heal itself and is part of the body's immune response. Signs of inflammation are swelling, heat, redness and pain.

Insulin is a peptide hormone produced in the pancreas. It is a most important hormone as it is central in regulating carbohydrate and fat metabolism. It produces glycogen from glucose and it turns excess glucose into body fat to store in adipose tissues whilst controlling the level of sugar in the blood. Insulin deficiency and insulin resistance create Diabetes 1 & 2.

Iodine is a mineral found in some foods such as sea vegetables, fish and shellfish as well as dairy products and grains. The body needs iodine to make thyroid hormones which control the body's metabolism and many other important functions.

Iron is an essential mineral in the body, and helps to make the red blood cells which carry oxygen round the body. The best food sources of iron include meat, liver, dark green vegetables, dried apricots, whole grains nuts and eggs. A drop in the required amount of iron in the body can lead to anaemia.

'J-K'

Kidneys are one of the most important organs in the body because they control the volume and cleanliness of the blood. They do that by filtering out the water soluble waste products produced by the metabolic processes and disposing of them in urine for excretion. The kidney regulates blood pressure by maintaining the salt and water balance and serves as a natural blood filter. The kidneys also produce hormones and enzyme called renin.

'L'

Lecithin is an important substance as it is the cornerstone of every body cell preventing the hardening of the cell membranes and keeping the cells healthy. Lecithin is produced to a degree in the major organs of the body such as the heart, kidney and liver. In food it is found in egg yolk, liver, meat and peanuts as well as whole grains and soybeans

Liver is a vital organ of the digestive system playing a range of important roles. Its main function is to convert harmful materials in the food we consume into harmless substances which are then filtered out and disposed of. Most importantly, the liver is essential in the regulation of cholesterol levels, synthesising it for transportation to other cells, as well as removing cholesterol from the body by converting it to bile salts for excretion.

'M'

Magnesium is an abundant mineral in the body. Hundreds of enzymes require magnesium to function. It is a cofactor in various biochemical reactions including protein synthesis, muscle and nerve function and blood glucose control. It plays a role in keeping a healthy immune system and building strong bones. Magnesium is available in fish, nuts and seeds, green vegetables, avocados, bananas and dairy products.

Margarine is a manufactured fat made from plant based polyunsaturated oils, such as sunflower, corn, soya and groundnut. The manufacturing process involves hydrogenation and other processes to make the oils solid at room temperature. Unfortunately, these also produce trans-fats which are considered to be harmful. Margarine contains a whole range of chemical residues from the manufacturing processes which are said to cause inflammation of the arterial walls.

Metabolism is a term that encompasses all the chemical reactions in the body that involves the production of energy in the form of heat from food.

Milk is said to be one of the most widely consumed foods. Normally, the first food we all consume is mother's milk, but milk can come from cows, goats, sheep, buffalo and other animals. Milk contains fat, protein and carbohydrate - in the form of lactose – in varying proportions. Milk is an important source of calcium besides many other nutrients.

Mineral elements are inorganic substances. The body needs them in small quantities for various different uses. For example, calcium and phosphorous for the formation of bones and teeth. Iron is essential for the formation of haemoglobin in red blood cells and also plays an important role in the immune system. Chromium is thought to enhance the action of insulin which controls blood glucose levels.

'N'

Nutrition - We are all familiar with the well-known saying "We are what we eat". Nutrition is the selection of food and its means of preparation so that when it is eaten, it can be utilised by the body. The choice of nutrition plays a vital role in bodily health.

Nuts are excellent sources of omega 3 fatty acids, high quality proteins, trace elements to help the hormonal functions in the body. They also provide good dietary fibre to assist with the rate of intestinal carbohydrate absorption.

'O'

Obesity arises when a human body contains an abnormally large amount of fat, that is, more than 20% over a person's ideal weight. Obesity can lead to an increased risk of ill health, notably type 2 diabetes, high blood pressure and heart disease.

Offal is made up of the internal organs of animals. Some of which, such as, the heart, kidney and liver are highly nutritious and delicious when well prepared.

Olive oil is a well-known mono-unsaturated fat, produced by pressing whole fresh olives, from trees mainly grown in Italy, Spain and Greece. It is widely used in cooking and salad dressings and it is a famed part of the much lauded Mediterranean diet.

Organic Food ingredients are considered organic if, in the case of plants, they were grown without the use of chemical fertilisers or pesticides, and in the case of animals, were reared without use of antibiotics, hormones or substances to enhance colour, flavour or preservation.

Oxidation is a combination of oxygen with a substance. This is what happens when iron rusts or when a freshly cut apple begins to change colour. When fuel burns, oxidation takes place and energy is produced in the form of heat and light. In the body, energy is produced in the form of heat when glucose, fat and amino acids oxidise. This process, sometimes, produces highly reactive unstable molecules called free radicals which attack stable molecules, turning them into free radicals also. Antioxidants, such as, vitamins C and E and beta-carotene can reduce the damage caused by free radicals.

'P'

Palm oil is an important and versatile oil and one of the most widely used in the world. It is 49% saturated 37% monounsaturated and only 9% polyunsaturated.

Pasteurisation is a heat process applied to some foods, mainly milk, fruit juices and beer. The purpose is to destroy any disease producing organisms present, thus making the product safe to consume.

Probiotics are live microorganisms which, when consumed in sufficient quantities, provide health benefits. Our digestive systems house over 400 bacterial species in the form of both 'good' and 'bad' bacteria. We need both but it is important to maintain the correct balance for optimal health. Diet, the environment, medication, especially antibiotics and even stress can change that balance in favour of the bad bacteria. To add to the good bacteria, probiotic foods such as yoghurt, miso soup, sauerkraut and green pickles can help to redress the balance.

Proteins - The protein we eat is broken down by the digestive juices into amino acids which are used by the body to make the specialised protein molecules needed to build, maintain and replace our various body tissues and blood. First class proteins are found in meat, fish eggs and dairy products whilst pulses, nuts and cereals are good sources of second class protein.

Pulses are pod grown edible seeds. All varieties of peas, beans and lentils are pulses. They are a vital source of protein for people who do not eat meat, fish or dairy products, but added to other sources of first class protein for meat eaters they can extend the more expensive ingredients adding extra flavour and thickening. Pulses also contain iron and fibre

'R'

Rice, like wheat, is one of the most important staple foods across the planet for human consumption. In Asia particularly it has been a food source for thousands of years. Rice is a complex carbohydrate and brown rice is the most nutritious as the milling process does away with the fibre and some of the nutrients. However, rice is often enriched after processing to replace them.

Rye - Technically a grass, rye is the hardiest grain grown the world over as a food stuff for both humans and animals as it tolerates different soils and climates well. It is used, either by itself or mixed with other flours, for baking bread in many parts of the world. On its own, it produces a very dark coloured bread, such as the well-known German Pumpernickel. As well as some protein, it contains calcium, iron, magnesium and vitamin B 6.

'S'

Sauerkraut is the German word for sour cabbage. It is, in fact, the fermentation of the cabbage which gives it its characteristically sour taste. Sauerkraut is eaten in many parts of Europe and is produced by finely slicing the cabbage and storing it, heavily salted, in large vessels, traditionally barrels. In time, lactic acid from the air causes the sugars in the cabbage to ferment and that, together with the salt, preserves it, giving it a long shelf-life. Like all fermented foods, it is probiotic.

Semolina is the course middlings of durum wheat. It is used in the making of pasta, breakfast cereals, puddings and couscous.

Sesame seeds are one of the oldest known oilseed crops. They are especially rich in the monounsaturated fatty acid, oleic acid. They are a good protein source providing fine quality amino acids with 100g of seeds giving 18g of protein. In addition they contain B vitamins as well as calcium, iron, manganese, zinc, magnesium and selenium. Sesame seed oil is used in salad dressings and dips and for frying certain food ingredients.

Smoked food - Smoking has been a way of preserving meat and fish for centuries. Other foods that are smoked include cheese, some vegetables, spices and, of course, the famous Lapsang Souchong tea. The food is exposed to the smoke from aromatic woods with vines or herbs for long periods at low temperatures. The chemicals in the smoke assist in the preservation of the food. Hot smoking includes heat in the process, taking a shorter time, it still imparts the characteristic and much enjoyed smoky flavour.

Sodium chloride is an ionic compound made up of half and half sodium and chloride. This mixture is common or table salt. It is used to flavour and preserve many foods. Salt is essential to life and the body has multiple mechanisms working together to regulate it. All scientists agree that a minimum quantity is required for survival, work continues to be done on the health implications of excessive salt intake.

Soya beans are widely used in food manufacture. They contain valuable protein and fat. They are mainly used as flour in cereals and milk substitutes. The oil pressed from the bean is used, among other things, to produce margarine.

Starch is a polysaccharide and the most commonly eaten carbohydrate. Made up of many molecules of glucose it is the most important energy store in plants. The far largest source in our diets is corn with wheat, potatoes, tapioca and rice also making up a big portion of our intake.

Sucrose is an organic compound made up from glucose and fructose and better known, simply, as sugar. It is a white, crystalline powder, produced from sugar cane or sugar beet. Sugar is widely used as a sweetener in food manufacture, in cooking and in food preservation.

'U'

Urine is a liquid waste product made up of excess water and water soluble wastes and toxins which the kidneys filter from the blood. Urine is excreted from the body via the urethra during the process called urination.

'V'

Vegetables are edible plants. They may be roots, such as potatoes, carrots, parsnips and turnips, or they may be leaves, such as cabbage and lettuce, flowers, like broccoli and cauliflower or, they may be fruit, such as, cucumbers and tomatoes. They are popular sources of starch and fibre and all contain vitamins and trace elements important to health.

Vinegar is a mixture of acetic acid and water and is used in cooking and in salad dressings to add a sharp flavour. It also has a use as a preservative of food.

Vitamins are organic compounds, which the body needs in limited amounts. There are two main types; water soluble and fat soluble. Although your body needs the fat soluble vitamins every day they are stored in the liver and fatty tissues so they do not have to be eaten every day whereas the water soluble vitamins are not stored and therefore need to be eaten more frequently. Following are some of the main vitamins our bodies need to stay healthy:

Vitamin A, this fat soluble vitamin is also referred to as Retinol. The most important sources of Vitamin A are: cod liver oil, egg yolk, liver and butter. Vitamin A is essential to good vision, skin health and bone growth.

Vitamin B1 is commonly known as Thiamin and is one of the water soluble group of B vitamins. It helps the body cells turn carbohydrate into energy. Found in most food ingredients, such as, cereals, nuts, seeds, eggs, beef, pork, liver and vegetables.

Vitamin B6 (pyridoxine) aids the body to use and store energy from proteins and carbohydrate. It is used in the regulation of mental function and the metabolism of homocysteine. B6 is found in fish, turkey, chicken, beef, pork, spinach, bananas and avocados

Vitamin B12 is obtained from food of animal sources. It is involved in the function of the brain and nervous system and the formation of blood

Vitamin C is a water soluble vitamin known also as ascorbic acid. It is an essential nutrient and a co-factor in at least eight enzymatic processes, for example, the biosynthesis of collagen. A naturally occurring organic compound vitamin C is a well-known antioxidant. It is available from citrus fruits, papaya, broccoli, Brussels sprouts, black currants, strawberries, cauliflower, spinach, kiwifruit, and red peppers. Deficiency in vitamin C can ultimately cause scurvy.

Vitamin D is a fat soluble group of vitamins. Strictly speaking it is not 'essential' as the body synthesises it when exposed to sunlight. It is used to regulate the absorption of calcium and phosphorous in our bones and to aid in cell to cell communication throughout the body. Food sources are oily fish, such as salmon, egg yolks, cheese, beef liver and fortified foods such as some dairy, cereals and fruit juices.

Vitamin E is the collective name for a group of ten fat-soluble compounds which are antioxidants. It stops the production of reactive oxygen species formed when fat undergoes oxidation. The best sources of vitamin E are wheat germ oil, sunflower oil, palm oil, olive oil, almonds and other nuts. It is also found in chili powder, kiwi fruit, papaya and broccoli.

Vitamin K is a group of structurally similar, fat-soluble vitamins that the human body needs for modification of certain proteins that are required for blood coagulation and in building bone and other tissue. It is also a protection against heart disease and it aids in optimising insulin levels. The most popular food sources for vitamin K are herbs, both dried and fresh, spinach, broccoli and Brussels sprouts.

'W'

Water is essential to maintain a healthy metabolic status. In an average person about 50 to 65% of their body weight will be water. That is around 40 litres. Water loss from the body occurs through the lungs, urine, perspiration and stools. It is replaced by drinking and from food. The amount that is required is carefully controlled in a healthy body.

Wheat is one of the most well-known cereals. It has many varieties. Flour milled from wheat is used, besides bread making, to produce a whole range of other products eaten today such as pasta, cakes and pastries. Wheat contains around 75% starch, 15% protein and some dietary fibre.

Wine - Many fruits and some vegetables can be used to make wine. However, the wine we are most accustomed to drinking is produced by the fermentation of grapes. Grapes contain both sugar and yeast so once the grapes are pressed and must is produced, the fermentation process can start. Fermentation ends when all the sugar is consumed or when the alcohol level is sufficiently high to stop yeast activity.

Y'

Yeast - By fermentation, yeast converts carbohydrates into carbon dioxide and alcohols so the most common uses of yeast take place in brewing and in baking. Yeast is a good source of vitamin B.

Yoghurt or Yogurt is produced by the bacterial fermentation of milk. These bacteria are known as yogurt cultures. Commercial yogurt often contains added sugar and fruit or other flavourings. Probiotic yogurt is also commercially available or can be homemade.

'Z'

Zinc is a very important essential trace element helping to stimulate the activity of 100 different enzymes. Zinc supports an effective immune system, properly synthesises DNA and plays a vital role in growth and healing injuries. Low levels of zinc make a person more susceptible to disease. Foods that contain zinc are, oysters and other shell fish, veal liver, meat, wheat germ, pumpkin seeds, cashew nuts, chocolate and cocoa.

G. I. BEKES 2014